MESMERISING THE BODY

MESMERISING THE BODY

A Study of Magical Anaesthetic Surgery in Colonial Bengal

Rajib Roson Ghosal

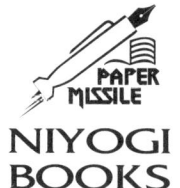

NIYOGI BOOKS

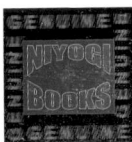

Published by
NIYOGI BOOKS
Block D, Building No. 77,
Okhla Industrial Area, Phase-I,
New Delhi-110 020, INDIA
Tel: 91-11-26816301, 26818960
Email: niyogibooks@gmail.com
Website: www.niyogibooksindia.com

Text © Rajib Roson Ghosal

Editor: Sucharita Ghosh
Design: Shashi Bhushan Prasad
Cover design: Pinaki De

ISBN: 978-81-992494-1-7
Publication: 2026

Every effort has been made to ensure the accuracy of the information presented in this book. The images used in this book come from either the public domain or from the public commons, unless otherwise stated.

All rights are reserved. No part of this publication may be reproduced or transmitted in any form or by any means, electronic or mechanical, including photocopying, recording or by any information storage and retrieval system without prior written permission and consent of the Publisher.

Printed at Niyogi Offset Pvt. Ltd., New Delhi, India

CONTENTS

Preface   7

Introduction   9

Forging a Path to Healing
*The Journey of Western Medicine in
Nineteenth-Century Calcutta (1830-1870)*   25

Traversing Wonders
*Historicizing the Mesmeric Anaesthetic Surgeries at the Calcutta
Mesmeric Hospital (November 1846 to September 1848)*   50

Descent of the Enigmatic Curtain
Exploring the Final Phase of Mesmerism—Challenges and Decline   120

Mesmerism's Legacies
*Power Dynamics, Cultural Exchange, and the Blurring
of Scientific and Non-Scientific Practices with Special Focus
on the Theosophical Society*   152

Conclusion   169

Endnotes   175

Appendices   189

Glossary   206

Selected Bibliography   207

Acknowledgements   216

Index   217

This study is about an invisible force with visible & tangible consequences ...

This study is about an undeniable science – Mesmerism.

PREFACE

This book delves into the fascinating history of mesmerism—a unique method for relieving surgical pain before the advent of ether or chloroform—in colonial Bengal. It embarks on an astonishing journey, unravelling the captivating social and historical dimensions surrounding this unique therapeutic method that once graced Bengal during the British era.

Navigating the labyrinth of historical sources, it has been revealed that while the threads of mesmeric surgery in medical practices are diverse and scattered, concrete traces of historical evidence remain elusive. Thus, the narrative unfolds with a judicious blend of deductive reasoning and circumstantial analysis. In this work, I have drawn upon a collection of published and unpublished records, including Parliamentary Papers, Medical Proceedings, Despatches (both from Bengal and India), and Bengal Government Reports on Administration, Medical Gazettes, Medical Journals, Census data, Ph.D. Thesis, and writings on the history of medicine. Yet, my endeavour does not merely rest upon readily available resources.

Drawing from an extensive array of official records and institutional documents, this volume integrates an exhaustive examination of medicinal practices that constituted a distinctive and unconventional method for inducing numbness during surgical procedures. There are notes providing detailed references for information presented. Additionally, a bibliography is appended at the conclusion of the text.

It is incumbent upon me to assert that the interpretations and opinions set forth in this book, along with any perceived limitations, rest solely within my purview.

I hope my endeavour will serve as a catalyst, inspiring further inquiries into the realms of colonial and contemporary India. Should this work succeed in eliciting sufficient interest, thought-provoking discussions, and fostering a fertile ground for related studies, I shall consider its purpose nobly fulfilled.

INTRODUCTION

The relentless pursuit of technological marvels and the resounding triumphs of medical science perpetually vie for supremacy. In the blink of an eye, once incurable afflictions are banished from the human form and, within mere seconds, a miraculous injection liberates the suffering patient from excruciating torment. But cast your gaze to a time when advanced technology, electrical wonders, and the comfort of chloroform remained elusive, and the plight of acute pain gripped patients mercilessly. It is an indisputable fact that surgery stands as an awe-inspiring testament to modern medical ingenuity. However, delve further into history, and encounter the extraordinary inception of amputation as a means to alleviate and heal, a revolutionary breakthrough that traces its origins back to the remarkable sage and physician Sushruta dating back to 600 BCE. Witness the audacious spirit of pioneers like Sushruta, whose indomitable pursuit of healing has left an indelible mark on the very fabric of medical progress.[1] French military doctor Ambroise Paré started modern surgical operations in the middle of the sixteenth century.[2] After him two men contributed further to the knowledge of modern surgery. They were John Hunter[3] and Philip Syng Physick.[4] But the idea of palliative or medical care to relieve physical pain during surgical operations was still an unimaginable thought since anaesthesia had not been discovered yet.

In 1842 Dr Robert Mortimer Glover first gave a comprehensive description of anaesthesia by testing the effect of chloroform on animals in his thesis. In 1838 he co-founded the Paris Medical Society and served as its first vice president. He won the Medical Society of London's Fothergill Gold Medal in 1846 for his lecture 'On the Pathology and Treatment of Scrofula', though he had not thought of using it on humans yet.[5] In contrast, using chloroform for anaesthetic surgery was successful and its comprehensive application was carried out by James Y. Simpson.[6] It must be mentioned here that before the invention of chloroform, multiple experiments like nitrous oxide or laughing gas, carbonic acid gas, sulphuric ether gas, animal magnetism or mesmerism, and ether gas were applied to numb the body.[7] Among these applications, at the beginning the most effective application for anaesthesia was mesmerism. During the middle of the nineteenth century, mesmerism played a vital role in continuing painless surgical operations.[8] This book is an attempt to depict the journey of painless surgery through mesmerism in colonial Bengal, with its success, responses and challenges. The study primarily focuses on the Calcutta

Mesmeric Hospital, delving into its historical significance, treatment methodologies, and impact on the development of mesmerism and alternative medical practices in the region during its operational period.

The Birth of Mesmerism

In the annals of history, the understanding of magnetism and its early proponents occupies a fascinating chapter. Around the year 1679, the distinguished continental physician Van Helmont demonstrated a notable grasp of magnetism, marking an early instance of its recognition.[9] However, attributions and discussions concerning the discovery of magnetism's principles have been a subject of debate. In this context, William Maxwell asserted that Franz Mesmer played a pivotal role in advancing Helmont's comprehension of magnetism.[10] This historical narrative takes us back to the history of magnetic therapy, tracing its origins to as far back as 600 BCE. The first documented encounter with a magnet is attributed to a young shepherd named Magnes who, while wandering the slopes of Mount Ida, observed the remarkable effects of a lodestone on his iron-tipped staff. It is from the shepherd's name, Magnes, that the term 'magnet' is believed to have derived. Another theory suggests that the word 'magnet' finds its origin in Magnesia, a region in Asia Minor where lodestones were plentifully discovered.[11] The ancient Egyptians referred to these magnetic stones as lodestones and harnessed their purported powers to enhance longevity and vitality.

Legendary stories even attribute Cleopatra with wearing a polished lodestone on her forehead, convinced that it contributed to her enduring youth and beauty. As we delve further into history, we find intriguing instances of early medical practitioners exploring the potential of magnetic therapy. In 46 CE, the physician Scribonius Largus recommended the use of electric torpedo fish to alleviate conditions like headaches and gouty arthritis. The ancient Romans similarly turned to magnetic therapy in the treatment of eye diseases.[12] Moving through time, we encounter figures like the French physician Marcel, who employed magnets to address headaches, and the Islamic physician Avicenna (980-1037) known for using magnetic treatments to combat depression among his patients. In more recent centuries, luminaries like Paracelsus (1493-1541), often regarded as the father of modern medicine, proposed that magnets possessed a force capable of influencing the vital life force within the body. These historical milestones in magnetic therapy lay the foundation for our contemporary understanding of this intriguing field.[13]

In 1778 in Paris, when Franz Anton Mesmer proved the existence of an invisible cosmic fluid passing through the living body, all the western countries were taken aback. It was when animistic, vitalistic and mechanistic theories developed. These theories describe the visible effects of invisible causes through scientific ways. In France, the Royal Commission was set up in 1784 by Louis XVI to investigate animal magnetism's process and treatment. It was named 'mesmerism' after the first successful application of animal magnetism by F.A. Mesmer.[14] Franz Anton Mesmer or Frederick Anthony Mesmer, born on 23 May 1734, in Switzerland, pursued a rigorous education in medicine in Vienna. In the year 1776, he made a significant contribution to the field by publishing a work exploring the influence of celestial bodies on the human body. Prior to this, in 1773, guided by the recommendation of the Jesuit father Maximilian Hell, a distinguished professor of Astronomy at Vienna, Mesmer reintroduced the therapeutic use of magnets to alleviate various maladies. Upon retiring to his native Switzerland, Mesmer's dedication to the welfare of the less privileged became evident. He demonstrated a profound belief in the efficacy of his chosen remedies. Mesmer developed a form of mass therapy in Paris, including rituals and equipment such as a *baquet*, a wooden vat filled with 'magnetised' water and 20 bent metal rods. He established the first *baquet* in an apartment of the Place Vendome with musical instruments. Manipulating the fluidum through magnetism, Mesmer aimed to re-establish the balance of this vital force, thereby treating a range of ailments, from hysteria and paralysis to blindness and epilepsy.[15] He passed away on 5 March 1815, in Merseburg.[16]

The year 1817 marked a pivotal moment in the history of mesmerism, as Prussian dominions instituted a substantial regulatory framework. This legislation confined the practice of mesmerism exclusively to the medical profession, attesting to its recognized potential within the realm of medicine. This legal demarcation ensured that mesmerism was administered and studied within a structured, professional context. Subsequently, in 1818, the Academy of Sciences in Berlin underscored the significance of mesmerism by offering a generous prize of 3340 francs for the most outstanding treatise on the subject. This prestigious award served as a compelling incentive, encouraging rigorous research and comprehensive documentation, thereby fostering a deeper comprehension of mesmerism's fundamental principles and practical applications.[17]

In the year 1825, M. Foissac for the first time proposed an influential experiment to the esteemed Academie de Medicine. He advocated the induction of a somnambulist—a person in a state of sleepwalking or trance induced by animal magnetism. The objective of this proposal was to afford members of the academy a first-hand encounter with the extraordinary phenomena associated with animal magnetism. This initiative vividly reflected the escalating interest and inquisitiveness surrounding mesmerism within both scientific and medical circles during the nineteenth century.[18] Though this neonate practice was discontinued due to political vengeance in contemporary France, in 1829 a Mesmerism Movement was started in England following the Irish doctor Richard Chenevix's visit to London.[19] The advent of mesmerism in the field of surgery marked a significant development in medical history, and its introduction in England is attributed to the pioneering efforts of John Elliotson in the year 1837. John Elliotson, a prominent physician and professor of medicine at University College London, played a pivotal role in popularizing and integrating mesmerism into the practice of surgery. His endeavours not only showcased the potential of mesmerism as an innovative therapeutic tool but also challenged established medical conventions. One notable account of these early mesmerism experiments can be traced back to the pages of the *London Medical and Physical Journal* in 1829. This publication served as a platform for the documentation and dissemination of the ground-breaking work conducted by Elliotson and his contemporaries. It provided a glimpse into the novel approaches being explored within the medical community, particularly with regard to the use of mesmerism as an adjunct to surgical procedures. Meanwhile James Braid, a surgeon from Manchester, became interested in mesmerism.[20] In 1843 he published a book on neuropsychology on the rationale of nervous sleep. Instead of the word mesmerism though, he liked to use the term 'hypnotism'.[21]

Mesmerism's Journey to the New World: Colonial India and America

The historical relationship between England, India and America has its origins in colonialism, a period marked by the expansion and influence of the British Empire. British colonial rule in India, spanning nearly two centuries, resulted in a rich exchange of ideas, languages and traditions, leaving a lasting impact on modern Indian society. In the case of America, early English colonisation and interactions with Native American cultures and African slaves contributed to a unique blend of traditions and norms, shaping American culture. The historical legacy of colonialism has evolved into a complex tapestry of cultural interactions that continues to influence the global landscape. Charles Poyen was a Frenchman who came to the United States in the early 1830s.[22] He had a background in mesmerism and was a proponent of Franz Mesmer's ideas, particularly the concept of 'animal magnetism'. Poyen believed that mesmerism could be used for various therapeutic and curative purposes. Upon his arrival in the United States, Poyen began giving lectures and demonstrations on mesmerism. He travelled extensively throughout the country, conducting public lectures and practical demonstrations to introduce Americans to the principles of mesmerism. Poyen wrote and published several books and pamphlets on mesmerism, including 'Mesmerism Revealed: The Facts and Philosophy of Mesmerism', which helped disseminate information about the practice and its potential benefits. Charles Poyen's work was instrumental in bringing mesmerism to the attention of the American public and medical community. While it's worth noting that mesmerism was met with scepticism and controversy in some quarters, Poyen's efforts helped lay the foundation for the study and exploration of mesmerism in the United States.[23] In subsequent years, mesmerism found its way to prominence in the United States, owing to the ardent efforts of several notable figures. Among these luminaries were A. Sidney, Dr Valentine Mott, who held the prestigious position of Professor of Surgery at Columbia College,[24] Francis Delafield, the inaugural president of the Association of American Physicians,[25] and John W. Francis, a distinguished physician and co-founder of the New York Academy of Medicine.[26] Furthermore, Dr Ackley, who served as a Professor of Medicine and Surgery at Cleveland Medical College, played a pivotal role in this process. Alongside these prominent names, a cadre of physicians, including Dr Bodinier, Dr Ducas, Dr Wheelock, and Dr Bostwick, actively contributed to the propagation and acceptance of mesmerism within the American medical community.[27]

Mesmerism reached India in 1845 with the arrival of the Scottish Civil Surgeon Dr James Esdaile. The East India Company appointed him in charge of Hooghly Imambarah Hospital or Hazi Muhammad Mohsin Hospital. Agha Muhammad Motahar, a Persian, arrived in India during the latter part of Emperor Aurangzeb's reign and established his trade in Hooghly, a thriving commercial port at the time. He eventually settled there permanently and founded an *imambarah*. This religious institution was later rebuilt and maintained by Muhammad Salch, also known as Salah Uddin Muhammad Khan. Hajee Faizu Uah, the nephew (sister's son) of Agha Muhammad Motahar, accompanied his uncle from Persia to India. After his uncle's passing, Faizu Uah married one of his uncle's widows named Zainab Khanum. Zainab had a daughter named Marium, also known as Mannoojan Khanum, from her previous marriage. Mannoojan entered into matrimony with Salahuddin and inherited the landed properties, including Pargana Syedpur, in Jessore (now in Khulna), which were left by her late husband. Faizu Uah and Zainab had a son named Muhammad Mohsin. Consequently, Muhammad Mohsin is considered a brother-in-law of Salahuddin Muhammad Khan, the original founder of the Hooghly Imambarah, as well as of Haji Muhammad Mohsin.[28] The Imambarah Hospital, primarily supported by the Mohsin Fund and private subscriptions from mills across the river, owes its existence to the dedicated efforts of Dr Thomas Alexander Wise, who served as the Civil Surgeon. Initially located in a rented house in Chawkbazar, and later in a property on Mogaltuli Lane, formerly a madrasa, the hospital was under Dr T.A. Wise's administration. In 1839, Dr Wise was succeeded by Dr James Esdaile.[29] The successful application of mesmerism in surgical procedures in Hooghly inspired British physician Joseph Johnson to similarly explore the practice of mesmerism in Madras. Dr Esdaile's pioneering work in mesmerism had a lasting impact, transcending geographical boundaries and influencing practitioners like Joseph Johnson.[30]

On 4 April 1845, J. Esdaile successfully performed his first painless surgical operation on a mesmerised patient in the Indian subcontinent at Hooghly Imambarah General Hospital. By 22 January 1846, Esdaile reported 103 cases of painless surgery through mesmeric anaesthesia. As a result of this success, the three successive governors of Bengal, Sir Herbert Maddock, The Marquis of Dalhousie, and Sir John Litter, publicly acknowledged its importance and encouraged its introduction in government hospitals. Esdaile was rewarded for introducing mesmerism in India. It was the first step in the establishment and progress of mesmerism in the Indian subcontinent.[31] Esdaile performed mesmeric surgery at Hooghly Imambarah Hospital, Hooghly Jail Hospital, Calcutta Mesmeric Hospital, and Sukeahs Lane Hospital & Dispensary.[32] He also published several articles in the *Calcutta Medical Journal*. He shared his experiences in the diary *Mesmerism in India and its Practical Application in Surgery and Medicine* (1846). Esdaile submitted the reports of his successful mesmeric surgery to the Calcutta Mesmeric Hospital Committee members H.M. Elliot, Esq., James Hume, Esq., Dr Martin, Rev. H. Fisher, Rev. Mr La Croix, Rajah Kali Krishna, Rajah Sutt Churn Ghosal, Rajah Pertub Chunder Sing, Baboo Ramgopal Ghose, and Baboo Rama Persaud Roy.[33]

The application of mesmeric anaesthesia was disrupted after the advent of ether gas and chloroform. The anti-mesmerists, Thomas Wakley and John Forbes, argued that the process of mesmerism was a time-consuming method and not suitable for emergency cases. However, on the other side, German physician Joseph Ennemoser claimed that mesmerism was much more preferable than ether gas as anaesthetics for the body. If the patient could not sleep by mesmerism, only then could ether gas be used. In the case of seriously ill and weak patients, anything could be tried to avoid using ether.[34] If one lists successful anaesthetic operations where ether was used, one can find out ether's harmful side effects. In fact, several patients died due to the side effects of ether. Even after several painless surgeries on mesmerised patients at the Calcutta Mesmeric Hospital, no favourable report was submitted to the government, so the hospital was closed down.[35] After that, in 1850, Esdaile was appointed as the superintendent to the Sukeahs Lane Hospital and Dispensary, Calcutta. He tried to merge the Sukeahs Lane Hospital and Calcutta Mesmeric Hospital, but this plan was not fulfilled. Therefore, the Sukeahs Lane Hospital was run independently.[36] Here, he continued mesmerism along with the ordinary practice of medicine until his return to Scotland in 1851, but this was not the end of mesmerism. On 8 August 1853, Dr James Esdaile submitted a memorial to the United States Congress. In it, he vehemently denied the assertion made by the United States Congress that painless surgery became feasible solely due to the discovery of ether anaesthesia. Dr Esdaile pointed out that long before the introduction of ether, painless surgery was already being practised through mesmerism. He emphasized that in his hospitals the use of mesmerism for painless surgery was as common as it later became in Europe with the use of chloroform. Additionally, he noted that he had personally performed nearly 300 significant surgical procedures using mesmerism during his tenure in India before returning two years ago.[37] Mesmeric anaesthesia was still used instead of ether to remove a breast in London on 26 April 1854 by W.J. Tubbs.[38] In 1874, J.F. Clarke, an eyewitness to mesmeric anaesthesia surgery, provided a concise description of this practice in his book titled *Autobiographical Recollections of the Medical Profession:*

> There is no chapter in the history of Medicine more astounding and bewildering than the episode of 1837-38, when for a time animal magnetism or mesmerism engrossed the attention of the Profession and the public. It was not a mere popular mania, like that of the 'brandy and salt' or the 'magnetic rings'; on the contrary, it engaged the minds of some of the greatest physiologists of the time, and its 'manifestations' were witnessed by philosophers, poets, literary men, and amateurs.[39]

Bibliographic Survey

Mesmerism played a significant role in the historical development of anaesthetic surgery. The English East India Company established a hospital dedicated to the application and experimentation of mesmeric anaesthesia in Calcutta, a venture of immense consequence in the annals of medical history. However, it is noteworthy that the concept of mesmeric anaesthesia remained somewhat esoteric and unfamiliar to the inhabitants of Bengal at the time. Consequently, the Mesmeric Hospital, despite its pivotal contributions, became colloquially known as the 'Jadoo Hospital' among the local populace, which translates to 'Magic Hospital' in English. Dr Esdaile was popularly known as 'Jadoowala' or magician among Bengal's populace. This nomenclature obscured the true nature and significance of mesmeric anaesthesia and, as a result, its impact was not extensively discussed or recognized in the subsequent regional discourse. Therefore, to glean insights into this historical episode, one must turn to various foreign literary sources. These sources encompass a wide array of materials, including books, magazines, correspondence, official government documents, and historical archives. By consulting these rich and diverse resources, individuals interested in exploring this particular subject matter can acquire a more comprehensive understanding of the role played by mesmerism in the history of anaesthetic surgery.

A valuable book on mesmerism is *Mesmerism in India and its Practical Application in Surgery and Medicine* (New York, 1851), written by Dr James Esdaile, where he has thoroughly analysed all the surgeries performed by mesmeric anaesthesia in Hooghly and Calcutta and recorded the list and experiences of the recovered patients. Another significant work is Chauncey Hare Townshend's *Facts in Mesmerism with Reasons for a Dispassionate Inquiry into It* (New York, 1841), where he analyses the reasons why mesmerism did not gain popularity despite having a practical application. He also gives detailed explanations of the physical and mental condition of the human body after anaesthesia by mesmerism. The book *Numerous Cases of Surgical Operation Without Pain in The Mesmeric State* (Philadelphia, 1843) has been written by John Elliotson, an eminent professor of medicine at the University of London. He had also published a reputed journal: *The Zoist: A Journal of Cerebral Physiology and Mesmerism and their Application to Human Welfare.* Through this journal, he had successfully kept a record of reports of surgical operations worldwide through mesmeric anaesthesia and the number of recoveries.

One of the most valuable books to know in detail about the mesmeric hospital in Calcutta is *Mesmerism in India* (London, 1849), edited by John Elliotson. The book contains official reports of the mesmeric hospital and experiences of the patients who have recovered from the surgery through mesmeric anaesthesia.

In addition to the abovementioned books there are several articles which help in identifying unexplored or under researched areas. Waltraud Ernst's 'Under the Influence in British India: Dr. James Esdaile and his Mesmeric Hospital in Calcutta, and its Critics' (1995) discusses the evolution of mesmerism and how far Esdaile was successful in its application. In 'Colonial Psychiatry, Magic and Religion: The Case of Mesmerism in India' (London, 2004) Ernst explains that for the common people, hypnosis became a form of magic. The Mesmeric Hospital of Calcutta began to be looked upon with wonder by the lower classes of Calcutta as the House of Magic or Jadoo Hospital.

'Parrhesia and Clinical Practice: A Case Study of Dr. Esdaile's Mesmeric Hospital in Hooghly' by Punnya Rajendran is a recently published paper (May 2021) that tries to explain mesmerism through the theory of Foucault's Parrhesia. 'Mesmerism and Surgery: A Strange Chapter in the History of Anaesthesia' by George Rosen is an important article to understand the gradual history of mesmerism in India from its beginning till the end.

Despite the success of mesmeric anaesthesia in enabling painless surgery no comprehensive work to date has delved into this remarkable application during the colonial period. The Mesmeric Hospital's eventual closure, despite its triumphs, only adds an air of mystique to the tale. Thus, driven by this enigmatic chasm, this book endeavours to illuminate the untrodden realms, weaving together the threads of history and knowledge to fill this resounding gap. As we delve deeper into the intricacies of mesmerism's influence, another enigma comes to the fore – an absence of discourse on its potential in treating neurological diseases and psychiatric disorders beyond its mesmerising impact in anaesthesia.

Forging a Path to Healing
The Journey of Western Medicine in Nineteenth-Century Calcutta (1830-1870)

In the nineteenth century Bengal was the thriving centre of British colonial India. As a result, it experienced a pervasive influx of Western influence. This went beyond mere alterations in physical appearance, language, or attire. Calcutta, the epicentre of Bengal, pulsated with vibrant energy as the intoxicating infusion of Western influence coursed through its veins, igniting a transformative crucible of cultural amalgamation and intellectual dynamism. According to Pratik Chakrabarti, colonial warfare in the seventeenth century and the consequent loss of lives due to diseases raised significant mercantilist concerns among European nations, resulting in mounting national debts. The expansion of eighteenth-century armies, accompanied by their substantial costs, imposed a significant economic burden, prompting increased taxation and the initiation of administrative rationalization and centralization by the British Army. Taxation for military and naval expenses escalated, leading to a twofold increase in average annual tax revenue in England during the Nine

Years War (1688–97) and further doubling during the War of Austrian Succession (1740–8), and the American War of Independence (1775). The number grew six times over the course of 123 years, from 1660 to 1783.[1] During this period, naval medical care lacked permanent institutions, relying instead on sick quarters scattered in colonial port cities which, while cost effective, lacked proper supervision and often relied on unlicensed providers. However, by the early nineteenth century, diseases ceased to be a major cause of mortality. The systematic development of medical care in the navy and army, including the growth of hospitals as institutions, enforced discipline and efficient medical care. This transformation was part of a broader process where medicine assumed a crucial administrative role, subjecting the human body to state control and discipline. The arrival and advancement of Western medical practices took root, primarily driven by the necessity to safeguard the health of the colonial army in India's tropical climate. The military hospital located within Calcutta's fort primarily served European soldiers and visiting sailors. The majority of the patients were enlisted soldiers, while higher-ranking officers typically received medical care through home visits by doctors. In 1757, during a visit to Calcutta, Dr Ives Edward, a navy surgeon and explorer, observed that the hospital in Calcutta treated soldiers from the ships who suffered from severe deficiency diseases like scurvy and bowel convulsions due to scurvy, likely linked to the consumption of muddy water from the Ganga.[2] In Ives's words,

During the rains, this rich and fertile country is quite covered by the Ganges, and converted as it were into a large pool of water. In the month of October, when the stagnated water begins to be exhaled by the heat of the sun, the air is then greatly polluted by the vapours' from the slime and mud left by the Ganges, and by the corruption of dead fish and other animals. Diseases then rage, attacking chiefly such as are lately arrived. Here, as in all other places, sickness is more frequent and fatal in some years than others. The distempers are fevers, of the remitting or intermitting kind: for though sometimes they may continue several days, without any perceptible remission, yet they have in general a great tendency to it, and are commonly accompanied with violent fits of rigors and shivering, and with discharges of bile upwards and downwards. If the season be very fickly, some are seized with a malignant fever, of which they soon die. The body is covered with blotches of a livid colour, and the corpse in a few hours turns quite black and corrupted. At this time fluxes prevail, which may be called bilious or putrid, the better to distinguish them from others which are accompanied with an inflammation of the bowels. In all diseases at Bengal, the lancet is cautiously to be used.[3]

Within one year (1756-1757) this hospital provided care to a total of 455 patients. Dr Edward noted the seasonal impact on health, indicating lower mortality rates among the Bengal squadrons during winter. During his visit, 180 men had succumbed to illnesses, a substantial portion of the overall deaths in various hospitals across India during Admiral Watson's command and shortly thereafter.[4] This intertwining of historical events shaped the critical kernel of Indian medical history. It encapsulates the struggle between Eastern and Western medicine, the colonial forces seeking to establish dominion, and the resurgence of traditional Indian medical practices. The landscape of Indian medicine witnessed a profound metamorphosis, setting the stage for the intricate and fascinating tapestry that unfolded in the last four decades of the nineteenth century.

India, renowned for its abundant biodiversity, offers a vast array of medicinal plants and herbs, providing a valuable resource base for the development of the pharmaceutical industry. This availability of raw materials serves as a robust foundation, enabling the utilisation of indigenous resources to produce medicines and drugs. The British capitalist mind needed more time to acquire this knowledge; as India's population grew and healthcare needs escalated, mounting demand for pharmaceutical products arose from the second half of the nineteenth century. In response, the pharmaceutical industry took strides, manufacturing a diverse range of drugs and medicines to address the healthcare requirements of the populace. A burgeoning demand swiftly took root in Bengal's medical market, drawing admiration from a vast multitude of eager buyers. Subsequently, the landscape of pharmaceuticals shifted as foreign advice and guidance catalysed the localization of drug production, giving birth to pioneering enterprises such as Bathgate and Co. (1811), Wilkinsons (1829), Buttokrishno Paul and Co. (1835), and W. Markillical and Co. at Khidirpur (1840). The British Chemical Works imported drugs from America to Bengal, while C. Ringer and Co. brought drugs from England and Germany. The Bengali babus took advantage of these new opportunities and became the owners of pharmaceutical workshops.[5] The allure of Western medicine transcended the bustling streets of Calcutta, radiating into the remotest villages, where revered allopathic doctors were held in awe akin to deities.[6]

Nineteenth-century Calcutta reflected the uprooting of the Unani and the indigenous Ayurvedic medical system and the establishment of strong roots of the Western medical system in Bengal. Calcutta was the first important trading centre of the British colony in India. Therefore, the Bengalis were the first to observe the stormy attacks of Westernization on Bengal's soil. In 1638, the British established the first commercial base at Hooghly with the approval of Shah Suja, son of Mughal Emperor Shah Jahan and Subedar of Bengal. During the reign of Mughal Emperor Aurangzeb (1658-1707), with the consent of the Governor of Bengal Shaista Khan, Mr William Hedges, the first governor of the East India Company in Bengal (1681-1683), was protected by the British Army. However, on 28 October 1686, Shaista Khan's army destroyed the British trading post, and the British merchants abandoned Bengal for fear of further attacks. In this context Jadunath Sarkar commented, 'It was Shaista Khan's task to put an end to this terror.'[7]

In 1689, Ibrahim Khan was appointed the Governor of Bengal by Aurangzeb, and he proposed to the British merchant Job Charnock to come to Bengal for trade. Charnock came to Bengal in 1690 and bought three villages—Sutanuti, Gobindpur and Kolikata—on the banks of the Hooghly from the local landlord Subarna Roy Chowdhury and named these three villages Kolikata. The British government got the approval for free trade from the Mughal ruler in return for an annual payment of three thousand rupees.[8] Finally, Western ideas established their first footprints in Calcutta. By the Regulating Act of 1773, Calcutta became the capital and centre of the East India Company. Even after 1858, during the direct rule of the British Government, Calcutta maintained the same position. The capital was shifted from Calcutta to Delhi in 1911 with the arrival of George V in India. So throughout the nineteenth century, Calcutta became an important centre for the fusion of East and West. We can see this trend in medical science as well.

Whispers of Early Remedies: India's Pre-Colonial Healing Pattern

Before plunging into the analysis of the topic covered in this chapter, it seems desirable to provide a brief overview of the traditional ancient Indian medicine. According to the Puranic writings, traditional Ayurvedic medicine was developed in India around 5000 BCE. This science was first imparted by Brahma to Daksha Prajapati, who then passed it on to Surya's son Ashwini Kumar Dwaya, from whom Lord Indra once more learnt Ayurveda. In order to understand Ayurveda, the renowned Bharadwaja Muni later dispatched his followers to Indra. Atreya, also known as Purnavasu, was one of these students.[9] Atreya, a historical figure, taught at Taxila University. One of the foundational texts of Ayurveda, the *Atre Samhita* or *Vela Samhita*, was also written by him. Additionally, he served as a physician of King Nagnajit of the Gandhara dynasty, as mentioned in the *Ramayana* and the *Mahabharata*. Charaka was most likely one of his followers. Kaniska, the Kushan king, had Charaka as his physician. His works, including the *Charaka Samhita*, expanded the field of Ayurvedic literature. Another of Devaraja Indra's disciples was the king of Kashi, Dhanvantari. He was allegedly born while the sea was being stirred. Sushruta was one of his six principal followers. Sushruta, a native of Kashi, invented surgery. His *Sushruta Samhita* marked the beginning of a new era for surgical care. Bimbisara of Magadha's physician was Jivaka. The *Kashyap Samhita* is his writing.[10]

Chakrapani Dutta, an Ayurvedic doctor hailing from the eleventh century, made medicines by blending minerals with juices from plants and animals.[11] Greek physician Hippocrates revolutionised contemporary medicine. He argued that all the causes of physical disease were concealed in nature and disproved the widely held belief that the initial ailment was brought on by the disembodied soul.[12] Later, the early development of Unani was inspired by Arab and Persian elaborations on Greek medical systems made by individuals like Ibn Sina and Al-Razi.[13] In the context of history, the origins of medicine can be traced back to the Indus Valley Civilization, specifically in the cities of Harappa and Mohenjo-Daro.[14] These ancient urban centres demonstrated a remarkable understanding of public health, exemplified by sophisticated drainage systems. Additionally, archaeological findings from these sites have revealed insights into therapeutic practices, including treatments for ailments such as arthritis. Within the Vedic age, deities assumed a pivotal role in the realm of medicine. Of particular significance were the twin deities known as Ashwini, revered as physicians. The *Rig Veda* contains references to remedies attributed to these ancient healers. The *Atharva Veda* introduces two distinct therapeutic methods: the recitation of magical verses and mantras, alongside the application of medicinal substances imbued with magical incantations.[15] Notably, the *Rig Veda* also offers praise for physicians like Rudra, Soma and Varuna, acknowledging their medical expertise. Concurrently, Ayurveda emerged as a transformative system in the history of medical science.[16]

In ancient times, practitioners of Ayurveda adhered to three fundamental principles: the identification of specific causes for diseases, an emphasis on natural aetiologies over supernatural origins, and the recognition of diverse treatment modalities. Subsequently, the collective contributions of Charak, Sushruta, and Bagbhatt, known as the *Vriddha Trayi*, or the Great Trinity, marked significant advancements in the realm of surgical knowledge.[17] Around the sixth century BCE, the emergence of Buddhism and Jainism as prominent rivals to Brahminism played a crucial role in the development of medical thought. Within the Buddhist scripture known as the *Vinaya Pitaka*, one of the *Tripitaka*'s three parts, various therapeutic measures are elucidated, offering valuable historical insights into medical practices. This text emphasizes the pivotal role of physicians, the administration of medicines by nurses, and the active participation of patients in the success of medical treatments. Notably, during this period, the royal physician Jivaka of Magadha played a significant role. Furthermore, Buddhist monks played a crucial role in disseminating the principles of Ayurvedic treatment beyond the borders of India.[18] In South India, Ayurvedic medicine was referred to as Siddha. Eminent figures such as Nagarjuna, an alchemist during the Kushan period, and Vagabhatta, who consolidated the content of *Charak Samhita* into eight volumes to create Astanga Ayurveda, contributed significantly to the advancement of Ayurvedic knowledge. Another notable figure, Dhanvantari, served as a renowned physician at the court of Vikramaditya during this epoch.[19]

The Gupta period was a prominent example of healthcare development. During the reign of Chandragupta II in 400 CE, Fa-Hien, a Chinese pilgrim, visited India. He visited Peshawar, Taxila, Mathura, Kannauj, Sravasti, Kapilavastu, Sarnath and many other places. Regarding the aspects of healthcare in the Gupta Empire, Fa-Hien says:

> The elders and gentry of the countries have instituted in their capitals free hospitals, and hither come all poor or helpless patients, orphans, widowers, and cripples. They are well taken care of, a doctor attends them, food and medicine being supplied according to their needs. They are all made quite comfortable, and when they are cured, they go away.[20]

Hospitals, complemented by provisions for sustenance, access to potable water, and a consistent supply of medicines, were prevalent along the highways in cities and villages. This infrastructure ensured timely assistance to travellers and the underserved. Notably, from 925 to 975, King Srichanda of southeastern Bengal employed two physicians, primarily to provide medical support to those working in Brahmin temples, underscoring the enduring significance of healthcare in ancient India.[21] The confluence of Greek-Arab and indigenous Indian medical practices in India can be traced back to the time of Muhammad's invasion. The text *Maden-Ush-Shifa Tibbe Sikender Shahi*, a medical treatise written by Mian Bhowa, a courtier of Sikandar Shah Lodi, records experiences of several Ayurveda practitioners.[22] Notably, numerous Ayurvedic texts were translated into Persian, enabling the dissemination of knowledge. Practitioners, known as *hakim*s in the Greek-Arab tradition and *vaidya*s or *kabiraj*s in the Ayurvedic tradition, sought to harmonize their medical methodologies. While *hakim*s emphasized the trihumoral hypothesis,[23] *vaidya*s recognized it for both diagnostic and therapeutic purposes.

Throughout the Sultanate era, Persian and Ayurvedic medicine received simultaneous patronage. Firuz Shah Tughlaq implemented a significant healthcare initiative by establishing a medical institution known as *Shifa-khana*. This institution was dedicated to providing medical care to the populace, and it employed a considerable number of physicians who administered free treatment to patients. Notably, essential medicines were made available to patients without charge and, in certain instances, provisions for food were also extended. To sustain the operation of this healthcare facility, the monarch allocated endowed villages for its financial upkeep.[24] Similarly, Mahmud Khalji, from a healthcare perspective, founded a substantial hospital in Mandu. This establishment was notably equipped with an extensive pharmaceutical storehouse, ensuring a ready supply of medicines. Moreover, comprehensive accommodations were arranged for patients during their recovery, and an additional section was designated for the care of mentally ill individuals. The fiscal requirements of this expansive healthcare institution were supported through state endowments.[25] Noteworthy instances include the private clinic initiated by the Greek physician Altamish during Alauddin Khalji's reign, as well as the recorded presence of seventy hospitals and 1200 physicians during the time of Muhammad bin Tughlaq. Several medical compendia were authored by physicians during this historical period. Notably, *Majmua-i-Ziae*, a prominent compilation, was assembled under the patronage of a member of Muhammad Tughlaq's court. This manuscript serves as a valuable resource for understanding the state of medical knowledge and practices during that era. Most significantly, it draws upon a synthesis of Arabic and Ayurvedic medical sources, thereby underscoring the significance of ancient medical traditions in shaping the medical landscape of the time.[26]

During the Mughal era, a period characterized by its cultural richness and imperial grandeur, the patronage of medical practitioners by Mughal emperors was a notable facet of courtly life. This practice evolved over successive reigns, reflecting varying degrees of royal interest in the medical sciences. During the illustrious Mughal era, a constellation of eminent healers adorned the imperial courts, their luminous contributions spanning generations of enlightened rule. Under the benevolent reign of Emperor Akbar, a staggering number of forty-two distinguished practitioners graced the court, their names etching history,[27] from Hakim Yusuf bin Muhammad in the time of Babar to the multifaceted talents of Maulana Muhammad Fazal, Hakim Abdur Razzaq, and the revered Hakim Bhairon. Emperor Jahangir's era, marked by nineteen dedicated physicians, witnessed the healing hands of Muqarrab Khan and Hakim Ali. In the opulent reign of Shah Jahan, a cohort of twenty-four medical luminaries, including Shaikh Muhammad Tahir and Hakim Ma'sum Shustari, illuminated the court with their wisdom. The era of Aurangzeb featured the specialization in ophthalmology by Hakim Sanjak. These distinguished practitioners adopted a comprehensive approach to medicine, leaving an indelible mark on the annals of Mughal medical history.[28] Multiple hospitals were established, where *hakim*s and *vaidya*s or *kabiraj*s worked in tandem. During the reign of Shah Jahan, a significant milestone in the realm of healthcare was achieved with the establishment of Darush-Shifa, a notable hospital situated in the city of Ahmedabad. At the helm of this medical institution, the distinguished Hakim Mir Muhammad Hasim was appointed as its chief administrator. This healthcare facility was distinctive in its approach, as it brought together a diverse cadre of medical practitioners, including experts in Unani and Ayurvedic medicine, alongside Greco-Arabic surgeons. The collaborative efforts of these medical professionals were directed towards the treatment and care of economically disadvantaged patients, reflecting a holistic and inclusive approach to healthcare delivery during the Mughal era. This integrated system of healthcare came to be known as Unani Tibb, a term which persisted in the pre-colonial medical landscape of Calcutta, serving a diverse demographic from impoverished individuals to landowning zamindars.[29]

Calcutta Chronicles: Arrival of Western Medicine in Bengal

Western medicine arrived in India with the advent of the European merchants. Francois Bernier, Niocolao Menace,

Johan Ovingto and other travellers were also notably responsible for developing Western medicine in India.[30] Initially, the British merchants considered the indigenous medical system and medicine as suitable for the Calcutta-centric environment. Early European merchants started translating Ayurvedic texts written in Sanskrit into English for the treatment of their soldiers and to gain a deeper understanding of the Indian medicine system. Europeans came to rely on Ayurvedic medicine, initially blaming environmental factors, mainly the scarcity and high cost of Western medicine. However, in keeping with their empire's expansion, they took the initiative to convert the Indian medical system in the European mould. According to Sujata Mukherjee,

> Nineteenth century Kolkata witnessed the growing patronage of Western medicine and gradual undermining of indigenous medical system by the colonial state. The British colonizer gradually developed a sense of ideological and medical superiority after discoveries made by science in the West. Western science and western medicine are regarded as superior enlightened, and rational. While India's medical traditions like indigenous medicine, folk medicine practices have become increasingly denigrated as inferior to traditional, backward, irrational, and 'others.' The Director of Public Instruction (DPI) in his annual report of 1859-60, observed that Calcutta Medical College, as a

representative of western medicine, had become more and more useful to the masses and would eventually supersede those 'legal homicides' the village Kavirajas.[31]

When Tradition and Innovation Embrace: A Brief Outline of the Advent of Western Medicine in Colonial Bengal

There was a visible drive for producing native doctors to reduce the burden on the Company's exchequer. As early as 1707, hospitals were built to maintain European health at Garstin Place, Calcutta.[32] In 1708 Captain Alexander Hamilton visited Calcutta. He recounted his experience in the book *A New Account of the East Indies*. About the hospital that he saw, he remarked, 'The Company has a pretty good Hospital at Calcutta, where many go in to undergo the Penance of Physick, but few come out to give Account of its Operation.'[33] Actually at that time the medicinal facilities fell short of fulfilling the basic requirements of the Europeans. The Battle of Plassey (1757) laid the political foundation for India's Western connection. By 1762, nineteen native doctors were recruited for taking care of the health of the European army in Bengal. The Bengal Medical Service was started in 1763. The service recruited forty surgeons in Calcutta. Training for the treatment of Europeans by allopathic methods of diagnosis and Western medicines was introduced by 1772. The Provincial Medical Board was formed in 1780. Two or three senior surgeons were appointed in each presidency. By 1785 this number had increased to 234 and 630 in 1824. In

1788, Governor-General Lord Cornwallis declared that if a practitioner had not been working in a military camp or hospital for at least two to three years, he would not be given civil employment.[34]

The first quarter of the nineteenth century was a new era of 'Western Medicine' and the introduction of 'Political Medicine'.[35] The Europeans adopted the concept of 'Environmental determinism'. Orientalists began a dramatic in-depth analysis of Indian medicine for the treatment of European soldiers. At the beginning of their acquaintance with indigenous medicine, the British continued to experiment in the laboratory on the one hand, and translated several books of medical science on the other hand. William Jones founded the Asiatic Society in Kolkata in 1784, an institution established so that the Europeans could learn about the ancient heritage of India. He also researched Indian medicinal plants and wrote *Botanical Observations on Selected Indian Plants* (1799). In the same field, John Clark wrote *Observations on the Diseases which prevail in the Long Voyages to Hot Countries* (1792). The Assistant-Surgeon of Calcutta General Hospital William Twining (1790–1835) conducted numerous post-mortem examinations which formed the basis of his two books, *Clinical Illustrations of the More Important Diseases of Bengal* (1832 and 1835) and *A Practical Account of the Epidemic Cholera* (1833), which is essentially an extract from the former publication, intended for the guidance of those suffering from cholera in Britain.[36] In section 43 of the Charter Act of 1813, one lakh rupees was allocated to spread education and science consciousness in India. But like the linguistic dispute, there was no word on whether the science would be Western or traditionally Indian. So at this time, in medical science, one coordination trend was maintained. The Calcutta Medical and Physical Society, established in March 1823, had two objectives. First, to collect original papers relating to discoveries in medicine and surgery, and second, to coordinate the branches associated with medicine, botany, and chemistry for the advancement of professional knowledge. In 1828, the Calcutta Society elected four Indians, Radhakanta Dev, Ram Comul Sen, Madhusudan Gupta, and Raja Krishna Bahadur, as its members, and they prepared four research papers on indigenous medicine.[37]

The East India Company established Native Medical Institutions (NMI) in 1824 to institutionalize the Indian medical system. NMI became the medium to apply the Western medical system with Ayurveda and Greek medical education in the vernacular language. Apart from NMI, Calcutta Sanskrit College and Calcutta Madrasa also started teaching this hybrid medical system through vernacular languages.[38] At this time, learning Ayurveda and Greek medicine was compulsory in order to study Western medicine. Until 1826, twenty students, irrespective of religion and caste, could study in this institution. Later, the number of seats was increased to fifty. A scholarship of Rs 8 was provided. All Western medical books such as ones on anatomy, surgery, physiology, etc., were translated from English to the vernacular languages. A hospital was established attached to the Sanskrit College in 1832 for the application of Western medicine. Before reaching the goal of anatomical dissection, preparatory psychological nurturing was done through introduction to zootomy of lower animals like goats and sheep, and handling of bones and skeletons. Sometimes human skeletons were examined during surgery education. Charaka, Sushruta and the theory of Bhaba Praksha on medicine began to be taught in Ayurvedic and indigenous medicine in 1827. NMI had four departments, namely Anatomy, Pharmacy, Medicine, and Surgery. The Medical Report of 1828 stated that the progress of medical class students in the study of medicine and anatomy was satisfactory. In 1832, eighty-four out of ninety-four patients were cured in the hospital affiliated with Sanskrit College.[39]

Transcending Boundaries: The Ascendance of Western Medical Mastery over Eastern Healing Traditions

However, this harmonious relationship between Indian Ayurvedic medicine and Western medicine did not last for a long time. In 1833 William Bentinck formed a committee to examine the progress of the Native Medical Institution and the teaching of indigenous systems of medicine in Bengal. The William Bentinck Committee, led by Dr John Grant as President and including members such as J.C.C. Sutherland, C.E. Trevelyan, Thomas Spens, Ram Comul Sen, and M.J. Bramley, proposed the imperative establishment of a medical college for the education of the indigenous population. This

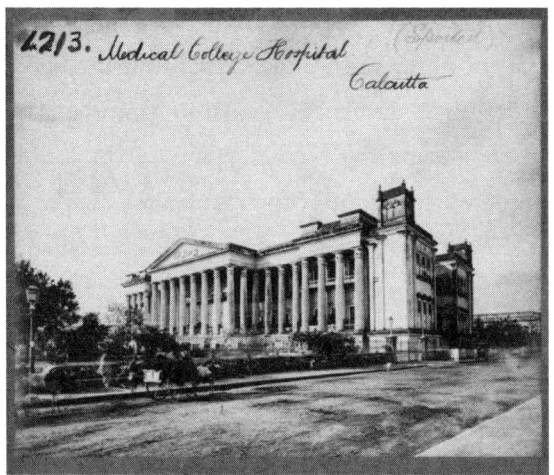

Medical College Hospital Calcutta, mid 19th century
Photo courtesy: Wikimedia Commons

committee submitted a comprehensive report on 20 October 1834, in which they strongly recommended that the state take the initiative to establish such a medical college.[40] As a result of the report, Calcutta Medical College (CMC) was set up to better Western medicine by breaking the relationship with indigenous medicine. At the same time, the Macaulay Minutes established a monopoly on Western languages in medical education. On the other hand, it was decided to shut down NMI instead of upgrading it. Similarly, medical education was discontinued at Sanskrit College and the Madrasa in Calcutta.[41] Although, Oriental thought sought to integrate Western medicine with the traditional Indian medical system, later on, imperialists began to characterize India as a backward country. So the way of Western medicine was adopted to bring Indians out of the darkness and lead them into the light of modernity. According to the imperialists, only the East India Company had this right and ability.[42] In the annals of medical education, a pivotal juncture materialized during the second year of 1836-37 when Dr M.J. Bramley, the esteemed principal of the Calcutta Medical College (CMC), meticulously crafted a novel syllabus. This revised curriculum, intriguingly, excluded the domains of Ayurvedic and Unani medicine, signifying a watershed moment in the institution's history. The courses that found prominence within this new pedagogical framework encompassed a spectrum of Western medical disciplines. These included the 'Practice of Physics', artfully instructed by Dr Goodeve, the 'Elements of Surgery', expounded by Dr Eggerton, and 'Chemistry and Pharmacy', under the tutelage of Dr W.B. O'Shaughnessy. Dr Wallich, an authority in botany, introduced students to the captivating world of 'Botany'. The subsequent year, spanning 1837-38, unveiled a curriculum characterized by a diverse array of medical subjects. These encompassed the domains of 'Anatomy and Physiology' led by Dr Goodeve, 'Demonstrations and Dissections' conducted by Dr R. O'Shaughnessy, and an exploration of 'Natural Philosophy and Steam Engine' guided by Dr W.B. O'Shaughnessy. Dr Wallich continued to impart insights into 'Structural Botany', while 'Operative Surgery' received elucidation from Dr Eggerton. The syllabus further featured 'Materia Medica' expounded by Dr W.B. O'Shaughnessy, 'Practice of Physics' by Dr Goodeve, 'Elementary Surgery' overseen by Dr Eggerton, and a unique opportunity for 'Clinical practice' at a hospital affiliated with the college. Noteworthy is the historic milestone that transpired on 10 January 1836, when four students of Calcutta Medical College namely Umacharan Set, Rajkrishna De, Dwaraknath Gupta, and Nabin Chandra Mitra performed the first dissection with the support of native demonstrator Madhusudan Gupta.[43] The legacy continued with Rajani Kanta Day conducting the second dissection on 28 October of the same year. Remarkably, in the brief span from 1837 to 1847, an astonishing tally of nearly 3500 dissections took place. Furthermore, the college became a hub of original research in basic sciences, yielding an impressive total of 537 books and articles.[44] A watershed moment occurred in 1845 when four Indian students from the Calcutta Medical College embarked on a journey to London for advanced studies at the University College of London. This endeavour proved to be an unqualified success, as these Indian students demonstrated their full capacity to compete with their English counterparts. This triumphant chapter in the institution's history underscored its pivotal role in advancing the cause of Western medical science in colonial Bengal.[45]

For the session 1847-48, CMC in its twelfth annual report stated, 'There is no Institution, connected with the physical or material welfare of the people of this land, whose success we have viewed with more unfeigned satisfaction than the Medical College of Bengal.'[46] From this time onwards, Western medicine gradually moved away from the path of integration with Indian traditional and Unani medicine. Between 1835 and 1858, Calcutta Medical College produced 456 native doctors. All of these native doctors were known as 'Licentiates in Medical and Surgery' (LMS) until the introduction of the Doctor of Medicine (MD) degree at the University of Calcutta in 1857. However, not all of them got jobs. Many also worked as family doctors of Indian regional kings, zamindars, or rich 'babus'. The Bengali LMS class of Calcutta Medical College was transferred to the newly opened Campbell Medical School, Sealdah in 1872.[47] The most significant changes in Western medicine in India took place between the 1860s and the 1890s. Structural and foundational administrative reforms were carried out in India after the Great Revolt of 1857. In 1858, Queen Victoria's Proclamation took over the Indian government's power from the East India Company. Now the British rulers adopted some initiatives in the Indian system of government and took several steps for social development, one of which was the change in medical science. Registration with the General Medical Council (GMC) was mandatory after 1858.[48] During this time, the British government was keen on advancing medical proficiency and medicine. In 1858 the British government passed the Medical Act. Soon after, the Medical College took the initiative to make a *Pharmacopoeia of India*, published in 1868 in London.

Two changes have been particularly striking in the medical system of Calcutta since this time. Firstly, an independent medical profession and, secondly, standardization of medicines. By 1842, six dispensaries had been established in Bengal. Their numbers increased rapidly in the following decades, reaching 255 by the end of 1879[49] and 500 in 1900.[50] Meanwhile, to develop the standard of medicine, the British Government took the initiative to establish a laboratory in Calcutta. William Brooke O'Shaughnessy compiled the *Bengal Pharmacopoeia* in 1844 to provide a guide to local alternatives to imported drugs and to facilitate the medical system. Initially, the British government provided expensive medicines to their army in the West, but emphasized indigenous medicine for the general public. Medicines to prevent local diseases played a unique role in developing the indigenous medical system. Dr O'Shaughnessy thought his job would be to prepare a class of native doctors for the future who were well versed in both English and the vernacular language. At the same time, they would use the knowledge gained from their own forefathers in modern Western medicine.[51] However, gradually, a special demand for Western medicine began to form in the 'babu' society of Calcutta. In addition to hospitals, physicians also practised in their private dispensaries. On the other hand, in the late nineteenth century, several hospitals were built in Calcutta, such as Eden Hospital in 1881-82, Ezra Hospital in 1887, Shyama Charan Laha Fye Hospital in 1891, and Shambhunath Pandit Hospital in Bhabanipur in 1897. In this way, the medical system of Calcutta was gradually Westernized.

The development of medical colleges in Calcutta and the rise of the English-educated middle class encouraged the middle-class society to develop two types of Bengali doctors. One, quack doctors with 'low-level employment' in rural areas, and the other, a class of doctors for English-educated 'babus' in urban areas. Registration of medical practitioners and doctors created a distinct difficulty for rural unregistered practitioners. The Western trademark gradually replaced the *kabiraj*'s fame with medical degrees. The historical trajectory of Calcutta's Bengali population reveals a profound transformation brought about by the forces of colonialism, imperialism and Westernization. In this evolving milieu, the emergence of a Calcutta-centric middle class, strongly influenced by Westernization, ushered in a momentous shift in the realm of medical science. The traditional practices of pre-colonial Kabiraji, Ayurvedic, and Unani medicine gradually waned under the pervasive influence of Western enlightenment. This Westernization initiative sought to infuse the Calcutta-centric 'babu' society with a contemporary ethos.

As a result of this societal shift, the denizens of Calcutta bore witness to a multitude of novel developments, experiments, and innovations from the Western world. Among these transformative encounters, a particularly remarkable phenomenon emerged – the integration of mesmerism into surgical practices to alleviate pain. For an extended period, painless surgery had remained an elusive aspiration. However, the introduction of mesmeric anaesthesia into surgical procedures offered patients the remarkable experience of undergoing surgery devoid of pain.

This pioneering approach engendered a novel paradigm in Western medicine, resonating deeply with both the 'babus' and the general populace of Calcutta.⁵² The fascinating journey of mesmerism, spanning from its origins in Europe to its eventual adoption in India, serves as a pivotal narrative thread in our exploration. In the forthcoming chapter, our endeavour is to delve into the intricacies of mesmerism, elucidating its underlying principles, mechanisms, and providing substantiated evidence of its effectiveness in medical practice.

Traversing Wonders
Historicizing the Mesmeric Anaesthetic Surgeries at the Calcutta Mesmeric Hospital (November 1846 to September 1848)

The ingrained knowledge that has been accumulated over hundreds of years does not silently welcome new revolutionary thoughts that could change the orthodox mindset of society. On the first broaching of any new branch of knowledge, there is a great commotion and combination among the old established school.[1] Mesmerism sought to establish its existence in the history of medical science and heralded a change. For a long time, the orthodox notion existed that there was only one path to cure a disease and that a patient has to endure acute pain during surgery. Dr Copland declared on behalf of the Royal Medical and Chirurgical Society of London, '... because pain is a wise provision of nature; and patients ought to suffer pain while their surgeon is operating; they are all the better for it, and recover better!'[2] It was not surprising that, against such a robust irrational notion, the emergence of mesmerism was welcomed by contemporary medical society, and the response was as expected. Contemporary physicians protested F.A. Mesmer's initial attempt to incorporate hypnotherapy into medical science. For this virtuous crime, Mesmer was rendered homeless and became an emigrant. Although he did not heed the shouts of this fierce protest, he gave a thumbs up to the orthodoxy of contemporary medical practice by giving hundreds of patients a sense of painlessness through hypnosis.[3] There was a time when the auditorium of his chambers became insufficient to manage the enormous number of patients. In continuing with the radiant light of Mesmer's success, Dr James Esdaile applied it for the first time on Indian soil at the Hooghly Imambarah Hospital. This chapter is divided into two conceptual categories, each comprising multiple sections. The first category explores the origins and historical trajectory of mesmerism, underscoring its significant contributions to medical science. The second category examines the early professional endeavours of Dr James Esdaile in India, notably his innovative use of mesmeric trance for painless surgery, with a special focus on the Calcutta Mesmeric Hospital.

Illuminating the Enigma: Mesmerism and Science

A traditional psychic and unscientific concept had continued since the beginning of hypnosis by F.A. Mesmer in France. It is sometimes recognized as associated with magic and sometimes with supernatural activity. Hypnosis and its applications in medical science began in India with the gradual expansion of Western medical science during the first century of colonial rule. However, mesmerism was applied to satisfy a unique need in contemporary medical science. Acute amputation pain during surgery was entirely relieved by the discovery of chloroform in 1860 and its successful application. However, before that, nitric acid, ether gas, and many other processes were experimentally applied for body fatigue, one of which was mesmerism. Mesmerism was the method that had been effective in relieving the patient from acute pain of surgery. Not only surgery related pain, but also the pain that comes with various diseases and illnesses was eradicated after the application of mesmerism. Mesmerism usually means a dormant state of the human body. The body becomes asleep and immobile, but the senses are active. Russia's Nobel Prize-winning physiologist Ivan Petrovich Pavlov commented that there was a difference between sleep and wakefulness with mesmerism. The human body's breathing process is normal during waking and hypnosis but decreases during sleep.[4] On the other hand, based on electrical waves received, fluency in the brain examined by Electroencephalograms or EEGs show how far the brain is active, even when the body's limbs are immobile under the influence of mesmerism. Hypnosis is not a miracle, nor is it magic. It is a scientific method that we are constantly experiencing. However, one is unconscious of it. One never thinks about how a child falls asleep listening to a humming voice while tapping his/her mother's hand. The same thing happens to us when we see a person's oscitation (yawning) or when we listen to an excellent and attractive speech; one's mind becomes detached from the thoughts of the outer world and only focuses on a discussion in a particular place. Also, one does not feel physical pain in any emotional state.

There are mainly four levels through which a person is taken to the stage of anaesthetic hypnosis. The first level is called Hypnoidal, where the body feels lazy. The limbs of the body gradually begin to feel heavy. The second level is called Lethargic State or Light Trance, where the body becomes completely relaxed, and the eyes gradually close. However, consciousness is still felt in all parts of the body. The third level is known as the Catalytic State or trance. It means going into deep sleep, but the unconscious thoughts of the mind become more assertive at this point, which begins to access the hidden part of the brain. At this stage, the hypnotized person begins to obey the orders of the hypnotist. The fourth level is called Somnambulism. It is the deepest level of the mesmeric process. The phenomenon of induced somnambulism, a key aspect of modern hypnotism, was first observed in 1784 by Puysegur at Busancy, coinciding with the year these records were documented. Puysegur emphasized that the essence of animal magnetism could be encapsulated in the phrase 'Believe and Will'. According to Puysegur, animal magnetism was not about the interaction between physical bodies, but rather the impact of thought on the body's vital principle [5] According to *The British and Foreign Medical Review*, Somnambulism is a condition in which certain senses and faculties are suppressed, or rendered thoroughly impassive, while others prevail in most unwonted exultation; in which an individual, though asleep, feels and acts most energetically, holding an anomalous species of communication with the external world, awake to objects of attention, and most profoundly torpid to things at the time indifferent; a condition respecting which, most commonly, the patient on awaking retains no recollection; but, on any relapse into which, a train of thought and feeling related to, and associated with, the antecedent paroxysm, will very often be developed.[6] The mesmeric theory is generally based on two main scientific concepts that have been already famous for centuries. The first was an invisible and unnatural force whose position was inevitable, such as the force of gravity, which kept the planets in their orbits, which could also be attributed to the liveliness of the living bodies of animals and humans. Another thing was the idea of treating disease by applying magnets. In the case of mesmerism, what is new is the relationship between the power of magnetism and the power of life. At the same time, the disease is cured by its application.

In addition to his achievements of in-depth knowledge of philosophy and theology, Mesmer revised and expanded his theories throughout his life, analysing fundamental principles of animal magnetism in his 1766 medical degree thesis titled, *Dissertatio Physico-Medica de Planetram in fluxu*. In this study, he talked about the effects of different planets on the human body, in which he laid the foundations of animal magnetism by giving multiple sources and proofs with justifications. He was mainly influenced by the work of Richard Mead (1673-1754), British physician and mechanical scientist, titled *De imperio solis ac lunae in corpora humana, et morbis inde oriundis* (1740; 'On the Effects of the Sun and Moon on the Human Body'). Richard Mead gave mechanical explanations for the usable energy behind physical activity and the diseases that resulted from it.[7] The same forces that create tides and keep the moon revolving around the earth could also affect the functioning of the human body. Mesmer introduced his book from the theoretical section, which began with the statement of Newton's Law of Universal Gravitation and Kepler's Law of Planetary Motion where he discusses the role of centrifugal forces and of gravitation in determining the orbit of the planet. Mesmer also used both Mead's medical theory and Newton's theory of gravitation to argue that energy of electricity is transmitted between minor liquid and solid particles of the body.

According to Mesmer, this energy is created by the action of body particles. These interact with each other, just as gravity does. The mass of the two planets, which makes the body a kind of battery, can create energy to animate itself. As Mesmer further developed his theories, he suggested that magnets are useful in treating disease, as the disease is caused by obstruction of this energy flow in the body, and magnets can affect this energy. Mesmer believed that the cause of the disease was the obstruction of the flow of energy through the body. Successful treatment is that which will be able to overcome this obstacle. Patients, by mesmerising treatment, try to restore the balance of the flow of nerve fluid in the body that was affected by the animal gravity force.[8] At first,

Mesmer treated patients by applying magnets to the affected part of their body. However, later, he realized that since all bodies produce these energies and the problem manifests an imbalance in the patient's body energy, he will apply animal magnetism with a magnetic stroke. According to Mesmer, there is only one disease and cure; by manipulating the secret fluid, Mesmer could put the patient in a state of peaceful sedation, which was likely an example of clinical hypnosis.[9]

In 1774 Mesmer learned to anaesthetize any object with a piece of the magnet from the famous physician named Maximilian Hell. After some experiments, Mesmer identified that anaesthesia could be possible without magnets. It was unavoidable that the contemporary society of physicians could not easily accept this ground-breaking change. Mesmer was expelled from Vienna by an orthodox society which still believed in traditional notions. He then came to Paris, where he enlisted the help of M. Delson, one of the most influential men of those times.

Mesmer established a clinic in France with the help of M. Delson. Surprisingly, countless patients flocked to his clinic instead of recognized medical centres. Knowing of his success, the French government sought to know the secrets of his medical practice, and they also wanted to recognize his medical practice. A Royal Commission was established by King Louis XVI of France, to examine the legitimacy of Mesmer's claims about animal magnetism. To this end, in 1784, Louis XVI formed a committee under this commission in which the members were the inventors of the guillotine machine: Dr Guillotine, scientist Benjamin Franklin, chemist Levsier, and others. Benjamin Franklin headed the committee, so it is often referred to as the Franklin Committee. Although the committee saw evidence of multiple successful treatments by Mesmer through animal magnetism, he could not break down the committee members' preconceived solid notions. So, to them, the treatment of mesmerism seemed unscientific. Meanwhile, Mesmer returned to Vienna when France's democratic revolutionary movement began. However, he was arrested on suspicion of being a supporter of the democratic revolutionary movement. Upon being released two months later, he moved to Switzerland.[10]

Trance of Transformation: Dr James Esdaile's Revolutionary Mesmeric Surgical Insight

Mesmer's animal magnetism did not disappear with him. In 1812, the Academy of Berlin in Germany started researching the same. Three years later, on 3 March 1815, Mesmer died. His death gave a new lease of life to contemporary research on animal magnetism. After his death, his ground-breaking discovery was carried forward by four pioneers. The Scottish surgeon James Braid coined the term 'hypnotism' in his unpublished 'Practical Essay on the Curative Agency of Neuro-Hypnotism' (1842) as an abbreviation for 'neuro-hypnotism', meaning 'sleep of the nerves',[11] later known as hypnosis in the 1880s. The second was Dr John Elliotson, president of the Royal Medical and Chirurgical Society. He discovered the stethoscope. He was the first to come up with an idea about the application of hypnosis in modern medical science. Evidence of successful treatment by mesmerism in various countries was successively published in a series called *The Zoist* by Elliotson. The third pioneer was Richard Chenevix, who spread the idea of mesmerism from Paris to London, and the fourth was Dr James Esdaile, who brought the idea of medical application of mesmerism from England to India. After the death of Mesmer, mesmeric anaesthesia became increasingly popular. Post Mesmer's death, mesmeric anaesthesia was first applied on 12 April 1829, by famous surgeon Jules Cloquet in Paris. He successfully removed a breast tumour by mesmerising a sixty-four-year-old woman named Madame Plantin.[12] In the same year, Richard Chenevix carried forward the anaesthetic process in England and applied it frequently. Also, in his report, he remarked, 'I was myself an unbeliever until my experiments undeceived me.'[13] He also noted that a special hospital for treatment was set up in Berlin, where mesmerism was applied in place of medicine. He mentions a total of 129 painless operations by mesmerism from 23 May 1828 to 20 January 1829, of which ninety-eight manifested undeniable effects. In the final part of his report, he said,

> ... however wonderful mesmerism may appear, one thing relating to it still more wonderful, that its truth has even been questioned; since it is in the power of everyone, without previous knowledge study, or acquirements, to

obtain a conviction at least in a week, perhaps in a few seconds. The truth which – Pythagoras told of the earth's motion reviled in its day, was reproduced by Copernicus two thousand years afterwards, and was again reviled; but this truth required all the mind of a Newton for its demonstration. To me the most extraordinary event in the whole history of the human science is that Mesmer could ever be doubted.[14]

The several successful operations by mesmeric anaesthesia attracted the attention of Dr John Elliotson. In 1821 he received his MD degree, and in 1831 he was appointed Professor of Medicine at the University of London. He was also the first to use the new instrument of auscultation (listening to sound/music from the heart), the stethoscope. He was appointed President of the Royal Medical and Chirurgical Society of London. One of his famous books is *The Principles and Practice of Medicine* (1844). One central focus of Dr Elliotson was to study the nervous phenomena, which led him to become an ardent student of mesmerism. He continued to apply mesmerism to his patients and maintained a considerable practice. In 1843, he published a report on the patients treated by mesmeric surgery. Many members of the Royal Medical and Chirurgical Society and others became receptive to the inestimable blessings of mesmerism. He also wrote the book entitled *Numerous Cases of Surgical Operation without Pain in the Mesmeric State*. Dr Elliotson requested Chenevix to perform mesmerising anaesthesia at St. Thomas Hospital. He also published the news of this success in the *London Medical and Physical Journal* in 1829. Another close friend of Elliotson also published a new journal named *The Lancet*. A series of reports on the scientific explanation of mesmerism in this journal was published by Elliotson from 1827 to 1828. However, a conspiracy was started by Robert Liston resulting in Elliotson discontinuing his publication with *The Lancet*. He then began to independently publish his own edited journal named *The Zoist: A Journal of Cerebral Physiology and Mesmerism, and Their Applications to Human Welfare*. This journal appeared quarterly from April 1843 to December 1855. A total of thirteen volumes were published. In this journal he published all the reports of successful, painless surgery on mesmerised bodies.[15] He not only published the mesmeric anaesthesia report but also provided the report of the hospital which was established for the application of mesmerism.[16] Thus, we get detailed information about the successful surgeries of London Mesmeric Infirmary in Bedford Square of London and other mesmeric hospitals in Europe, such as in Bristol, Dublin and Exeter.

Dr James Esdaile's seminal contribution to painless surgery in India commenced on 4 April 1845, culminating in the establishment of the remarkably successful Calcutta Mesmeric Hospital located at Motts Lane. Although the hospital's existence was relatively brief, its impact was truly remarkable. Furthermore, historical resources such as *The*

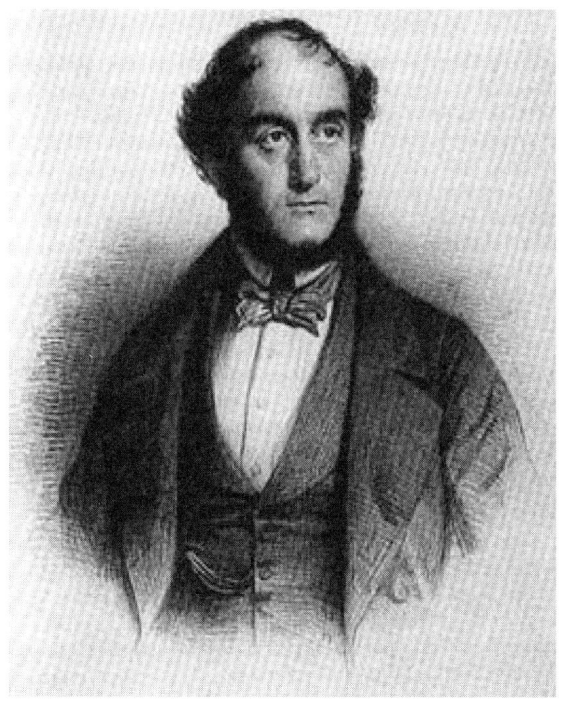

Dr James Esdaile
Photo courtesy: https://www.psychologytoday.com/gb

Zoist's article, Dr James Esdaile's memoir, and his other literary works provide invaluable insights into the inception of mesmerism in India and the captivating history of painless surgical procedures facilitated through mesmerism. In addition to these primary sources, archival records of the Calcutta Mesmeric Hospital, contemporaneous newspapers, and reports from the Department of Health and Family Welfare serve as vital resources for deepening one's understanding of the mesmerism movement in India. A meticulous analysis of this comprehensive evidence allows for a profound exploration of the experiences of patients who underwent transformative recoveries through painless surgeries utilizing mesmeric anaesthesia at the inaugural Calcutta Mesmeric Hospital.[17] The application of mesmeric anaesthesia to Indian medical science dates back to the arrival of Dr James Esdaile on Indian soil.[18] He arrived in India in 1830 and returned to Britain in 1851. For the convenience of discussion, his total tenure in India is divided into four parts. The first part was from 1830 to November 1839 when he was appointed Civil Surgeon in India on behalf of the East India Company until he retired due to an illness. He then went on a long trip to revive his health and returned to Calcutta in 1839. The second part was from the time he took charge of the Hooghly Imambarah General Hospital and Jail Hospital in November 1839 until the first mesmeric surgery was performed on 4 April 1845. The third period began in 1845 and lasted till 1848. During this time, lots of successful painless surgeries were performed through mesmeric trance by Esdaile. These cases were submitted as evidence to the Mesmeric Surgery Research Committee formed by the Deputy Governor of Bengal. The last period, from November 1848 until his return in 1851, was when he continued to apply mesmerism entirely in medical practice as the head of the Calcutta Mesmeric Hospital. This present research focuses on the third and fourth part of his triumphant journey to India although some attention will be given to the history of the first two parts.

Beneath the Mesmeric Veil: Chronicles of Painless Surgery by Dr James Esdaile at Hooghly Jail Hospital and Imambarah General Hospital

Dr James Esdaile was a Scottish surgeon. His research work was on *De Narcotics* ('On Narcotics') in his MD from the University of Edinburgh in 1829. In 1830 at the age of twenty-two, he was appointed as Civil Assistant Surgeon to the East India Company. Later, on 10 February 1831, he joined as a Military Assistant Surgeon. However, he suffered from asthma and bronchitis. Also, his lungs, in particular, were diagnosed as 'delicate'. Based on his medical report he was instructed to live in a warmer climate. Through his job, he not only obtained an appointment in British India that ensured his health requirement to antagonistic change from his home climate but also a lucrative career in the East India Company's service in India.[19] While serving as a military and civil surgeon at Azamgarh in 1835, he suddenly became very ill, and his health deteriorated. He appointed Assistant Surgeon R. Christie in his place on 27 May 1835 and took a short break from physician life.[20] He then went on a long trip, visiting Egypt and Italy. He wrote about his experience in his book *Letters from the Red Sea, Egypt, and the Continent*. He returned to Calcutta in November 1839. The East India Company appointed him the Civil Surgeon of Hooghly Imambarah General Hospital. At the same time, Dr James Esdaile took charge of Hooghly Jail Hospital from November 1839 to December 1841.

It will be helpful to understand the mesmeric surgical operations that were performed by Dr Esdaile by classifying them into two parts. The first phase was prior to the founding of the Calcutta Mesmeric Hospital, and the second period was subsequent to its founding. He joined the Imambarah General Hospital as a surgeon in November 1839, and he performed his duty as usual until 4 April 1845. On this day, he performed the first painless surgery through a mesmeric trance. He persisted until 22 January 1846, when he completed seventy-three painless procedures and reported his findings to the government authorities. However, the administration provided no helpful answers. Dr Esdaile thereafter continued his mesmerising technique until 31 July 1846. He carried out 102 painless procedures in all. A committee was established at the time by the Bengal government. It was to review the surgeries conducted by Dr Esdaile. He operated on ten patients, three of whom had to be excluded as they incurred fever so that ultimately only seven patients participated. The Calcutta Mesmeric Hospital was created following the committee's favourable recommendation in November 1846, and Dr Esdaile performed a total of 261 painless operations until this hospital building was razed to the ground in 1848 on order by Lord Dalhousie. Dr James Esdaile thus performed a total of 109 painless surgeries through mesmeric trance at the Imambarah General Hospital and the Hooghly Jail Hospital prior to the establishment of this exceptional experimental hospital in Calcutta. In our subsequent discourse, we shall engage in a rigorous examination of the surgical procedures performed sans pain under the auspices of James Esdale's mesmerism, with a particular focus on the efficacy and paradigmatic significance of this innovative approach to pain management in a clinical context.

April 1845 marks the beginning of painless surgery by mesmeric anaesthesia in India. Before that, Dr Esdaile simultaneously performed duties as a surgeon at the Hooghly Imambarah General Hospital and the Hooghly Jail Hospital. He continued his work as usual until he met Madhav Keora (Madhab Keora). The horrendous agony of double hydrocele made life even more miserable for hog dealer Madhab Keora than his seven-year prison sentence. The intense pain of this disease crippled this strong-looking man. He was sent from jail to the charity hospital to get relief from severe pain. This is where Dr Esdaile first saw Madhab. His pain worsened when the general hospital doctor started his treatment with the injection process. Describing the pain in detail, Esdaile says,

> The water was drawn off one side of the scrotum, and two drachms of the usual cor. sub. injection were thrown in. On feeling the pain from the injection, he threw his head over the back of the chair, and pressed his hands along the course of the spermatic cords, closing his eyelids firmly, and making the grimaces of a man in pain. Seeing him suffering in this way, I turned to the native sub-assistant surgeon, an eleve of the medical college, and asked him if he had ever seen Mesmerism? He said that he had seen it tried at the medical college, but without effect. Upon which I remarked, 'I have a great mind to try it on this man, but as I never saw it practised, and know it only from

reading, I shall probably not succeed.' He (Madhab) was ordered to remain quiet, and the passes were continued for a quarter of an hour longer ... The same process was persevered in, and in about an hour he began to gape, said he must sleep, that his senses were gone; and his replies became incoherent. He opened his eyes, when ordered, but said he only saw smoke, and could distinguish no one: his eyes were quite lustreless, and the lids were opened heavily. All appearance of pain now disappeared; his hands were crossed on his breast, instead of being pressed on the groins, and his countenance showed the most perfect repose.

Then, he was awakened by the native doctor Muhammad Ali upon returning to the jail. Madhab expressed his feelings in response to Dr Esdaile's questions. Such as ...

'How do you feel?' - 'Very well.' 'Any pain in the throat, or elsewhere? - 'A little uneasiness in the throat, no pain anywhere else.' 'What has happened to you to-day?'- 'I went in the morning to the Imbarah Hospital, to get the water taken out of my scrotum.' 'Was the water drawn off?' - 'Yes.' 'What do you remember after the operation?' - (Replied) 'I went to sleep soon after, and remember nothing else.' 'Did you eat or drink after the operation?' - 'I felt thirsty, but got nothing to drink till Kurreem Ali, the native doctor, awoke me.' 'Did anybody prick, or burn you?' - 'No, no.' 'Did you smell anything disagreeable?' – 'No.' 'Were you happy when asleep?' – 'Very.' 'Did you hear anything when you were asleep?' – 'I heard voices, but did not understand them.' 'Did you see any gentleman in the hospital but me?' – 'No.' 'Did you feel any pain in the scrotum after going to sleep?' – 'I felt none till I awoke.' 'Any pain in that part now?' – 'A very little.'[21] [Note: The above conversations were reported and signed by Mr. F. W. Russell, the judge, and Mr. D. J. Money, the collector, Budden Chunder Chowdaree Subsistent surgeon]

After that, Esdaile enlarged his mesmeric grounding based on textual knowledge.[22] Madhab was gradually taken to the 'somnambulism stage'[23] of anaesthesia. After giving continuous passes nearly three quarters of an hour, there seemed to be no pain in the scrotum. Even the pricking of his body with a pin did not restore his senses or wake him. While before, a slight touch of the scrotum was painful, after he was mesmerised, even pricking caused no pain.

The successful medical experience of Madhab Keora inspired Esdaile to start a new chapter in Western medicine. From that point onwards, he started using mesmeric anaesthesia to provide pain-free treatment to several patients, and was successful.[24] In 1845 many surgical operations were performed. All the operations were of an important nature. Among them the following are paraphrased accounts of significant examples of incorporating mesmeric anaesthesia:

On 7 April, Janokee-Sing (Janaki Singh) a stout looking peon, had sloughed off the whole scrotum from the effects of a hernia. The pain was most severe when treated with tamarind leaves. He did not sleep a single day from the time he arrived at the hospital till 15 April. From 15 April to 19 April, mesmeric anaesthesia was applied to him and his pain subsided.[25]

On 20 April Dr Esdaile reported:

> Jeolal, my washerman, aged 35, has been eighteen months ill; first with dysentery, afterwards with rheumatic fever, in consequence of which his left knee is bent upon the thigh at a right angle. I considered him to be a hopeless cripple. I mesmerised him to-day in a quarter of an hour. At first, he supported his knee with both hands; but soon allowed me to remove them, and suspend them in the air. The leg was then gradually extended, and straightened to a considerable extent, without awaking him. On June 22nd, His leg is now quite straight, and the knee flexible; he has got a violent colic, and when speaking to me fell down in a fainting state. Ordered to be mesmerised. On June 23rd He slept for an hour, and awoke much relieved yesterday; but a paroxysm returned last night, and still continues.— Repeat the Mesmerism. June 24th He remained three hours in the mesmeric sleep yesterday, and awoke quite well, and continues so. His leg is now quite strong, and he has returned to his work.[26]

Kangalee (Kangalay), a peasant, was frail and emaciated at eleven in the morning on 20 April. He suffered a fever four years ago and, as a result, sores appeared in numerous places on his body, leaving behind big cicatrices that resembled burns. One was the left elbow joint, which had been flexed almost constantly to the right angle for seven months. After twenty minutes of catalepsies, a bottle was placed beneath his elbow as a fulcrum, and the arm was gradually extended by pressing the hand. His muscles occasionally tightened up when he moved a little, but they immediately melted under Dr Esdaile's fingers and he continued to sleep with his arm absolutely straight and extended in the air. At two in the afternoon he awoke. He saw his arm was straight, as usually he knew not how it was done, had no pain, and could move it freely. On 2 May he pulled the *punkah*[27] daily with his left arm, for exercise. On 14 June he was released as cured.[28]

On 3 May, Bissumber Chowdry (Viswambhar Chowdhury) arrived at the hospital with bladder rupture due to retention of urine for three days. On 4 May, by mesmerism, he slept for two hours and, on waking, passed urine freely and felt a pain-free moment.[29] From 4 May to 11 May, Deno (Dinu), a prisoner, endured torment, after which he was released from torment by mesmerism.[30] On 5 May, Rantoonee Buttachargie (Ratan Bhattacharya), a Brahmin, who was affected by fungus haematites was cured painlessly by a mesmeric trance.[31]

On 11 May, Dr Esdaile reported,

Meeroolla, a policeman; aged 28, strong and healthy looking. He has got a fatty tumour of the right mamma, which he begged me to remove to-day. I desired him to lie down, and let me carefully examine it, and commenced mesmerising him. In ten minutes he was fast asleep; in five minutes more I transfixed the tumour with a hook, drew it up off the muscles, and cut it out, without disturbing him in the least, and he did not awake till half an hour afterwards. He declares that he felt no pain till he awoke, and remembers nothing after my hands were placed on his stomach, which was in about five minutes from the commencement.[32]

On 14 May, Dr James Esdaile conducted an initial consultation with Maduh, a robust-appearing *coolie* or porter aged thirty, at 11 in the morning. The patient presented with a chronic ulcer on his heel, persisting for two years, characterized by a thickened skin layer (approximately 0.5 inches) detached from the underlying tissue, necessitating excision. Following induction of mesmerism, Esdaile temporarily left the hospital to engage in a professional encounter in Chinsurah, where he was introduced to Reverend Mr Banergie, who expressed interest in observing a patient under mesmeric influence. Esdaile expressed reservations about exploiting this potent technique for mere curiosity but offered to showcase the patient, already under hypnosis, upon his return to the hospital. Upon re-entry, Esdaile was joined by Reverend Mr Fisher, Mr Banergie, and Mr Money, the collector, and proceeded to surgically remove the thickened skin from the plantar fascia, a challenging procedure due to its exceptional thickness and hardness, akin to a horse's hoof. Notably, Maduh remained completely anaesthetized throughout the procedure and for an additional quarter hour post-operation.[33] On 22 May, Mr T.M. Clermont, headmaster of the Lower School and Hooghly College, who had been suffering from a nervous headache was mesmerised in the presence of two Medical College students, Mr Philips and Mr Scott, Baron Law de Clapernou, the Governor of Chandernagore, Mr Russell, the judge, Mr Wauchope, the magistrate, J. St. Pourcain, and Esq., Mr Clint, Principal of Hooghly College.[34]

Mr Fisher sent a report to Dr Esdaile on the therapeutic regimen employed for Nazir Mahomed, a prisoner, on 24 May. Nazir had experienced acute conjunctivitis for the preceding four days, manifesting as a prominent vascular ring around the cornea, persistent lacrimation, cephalgia affecting the left hemcranium, and significantly impaired visual acuity, rendering him unable to discern objects with clarity.

Mr Fisher's report was as follows:

> On Saturday last, the 24th inst., I visited the Jail Hospital, in company with Dr. Esdaile, for the purpose of seeing a prisoner awakened out of the mesmeric trance, who had been suffering for some time from an inflamed eye. Upon our arrival the man was awake, and no further experiment

could therefore be tried with this patient. Another, however, immediately presented himself, who had never been subjected to the mesmeric influence before, and whom, I believe, the doctor had never seen. He had been suffering much for some days from severe pains in the head and face; though not at that moment in pain, it was thought advisable to try the effects of Mesmerism as a preventive. The manipulations were immediately commenced, and in seven minutes the man was in a cataleptic state. We tried various means to test the intensity of the trance: his limbs rigidly maintained themselves in any posture in which Dr. Esdaile chose to place them; and at last he was raised upon his feet; his back being slightly bent, his arms stretched over head, which was drooping upon his shoulder, and he remained fixed in this constrained position for some time, without exhibiting any symptoms of consciousness, or uneasiness. After a few minutes he was left to his deep repose, reclined upon the ground; and I understand that, since this first trial, he has never had the slightest return of the pains of which he previously complained: we were much astonished at the phenomena exhibited on this occasion; the limbs being so extraordinarily supple, and at the same time capable of being so rigidly fixed in any position, at the will of the operator. (Signed) F. Fisher. Chinsurah, May 29th, 1845.[35]

On 29 May, Dr James Esdaile reported a case involving Sibehurn Sing, a young and physically robust individual, who had suffered a traumatic injury to his thumb fourteen days prior. The patient's thumb had been nearly severed by a sword and, despite initial attempts to repair the damage, the wound had failed to heal properly. The distal portion of the thumb had become a source of discomfort and impeded normal function. Dr Esdaile successfully induced a state of mesmerism in the patient within a span of ten minutes, rendering him insensible to pain. Subsequently, Dr Esdaile performed a surgical amputation of the distal thumb segment, completing the procedure without awakening the patient. He soon after quietly opened his eyes, and Dr Esdaile asked him,

> 'Have you been asleep?' 'Yes.' 'Have you any pain?' 'No.' 'Has anything hurt you to-day?' 'No.' 'Do you wish your nail cut off?' 'Yes.' 'Look at it.' He did so, looked confounded, and exclaimed, 'It's gone!' 'Who did it?' 'God knows.' 'How did it happen, has it fallen off itself?' 'I can't tell—I know nothing about it.'[36]

In the case of Modoomohun Ray (Madan Mohan Roy), a twelve-year-old male patient was admitted to the hospital on 30 May with a compound fracture of both forearm bones. The wound had developed purulent matter, necessitating surgical enlargement. To alleviate the patient's apprehension, Dr Esdaile employed a calming technique, covering his eyes with a damp cloth. Unnoticed by the patient, Dr Esdaile successfully induced a mesmerised state within ten minutes, enabling the surgical procedure to be performed without causing distress. Upon returning three hours later, Dr Esdaile found the patient still asleep. Upon awakening, the patient reported reduced pain and no recollection of discomfort during the procedure. This case demonstrates the effective use of mesmerism in managing pain and anxiety in a paediatric patient undergoing surgical intervention.[37] A remarkable case study pertains to a forty-year-old peasant, Teencowrie Paulit, who presented at Esdaile's Hospital on 3 June with a two-year history of a maxillary antrum tumour. The tumour had precipitated a series of debilitating symptoms, including orbital displacement, nasal obstruction, pharyngeal encroachment, and cervical lymphadenopathy. Following induction into a cataleptic state via mesmerism, Dr Esdaile performed a protracted and intricate surgical procedure, notable for its complexity and duration. Throughout the operation, the patient remained utterly insensible, exemplifying the efficacy of mesmerism in mitigating pain and anxiety in surgical contexts. This case study underscores the potential of mesmerism as a valuable adjunct in surgical interventions, warranting further investigation into its applications in pain management. Here is the excerpt of the details of mesmeric painless surgery of Teencowrie Paulit as reported by Dr Esdaile,

> I put a long knife in at the corner of his mouth, and brought the point out over the cheek-bone, dividing the parts between; from this, I pushed it through the skin at

the inner corner of the eye, and dissected the cheek back to the nose. The pressure of the tumour had caused the absorption of the anterior wall of the antrum, and on pressing my fingers between it and the bones, it burst, and a shocking gush of blood, and brain-like matter, followed. The tumour extended as far as my fingers could reach under the orbit and cheek-bone, and passed into the gullet—having destroyed the bones and partition of the nose. No one touched the man, and I turned his head into any position I desired, without resistance, and there it remained till I wished to move it again: when the blood accumulated, I bent his head forward, and it ran from his mouth as if from a leaden spout. The man never moved, nor showed any signs of life, except an occasional indistinct moan; but when I threw back his head, and passed my fingers into his throat to detach the mass in that direction, the stream of blood was directed into his wind-pipe, and some instinctive effort became necessary for existence; he therefore coughed, and leaned forward, to get rid of the blood; and I supposed that he then awoke. The operation was by this time finished, and he was laid on the floor to have his face sewed up, and while this was doing, he for the first time opened his eyes... On 6th June he (Teencowrie) was out of all danger, and can speak plainly: he declares most positively, that he knew nothing... Here is a translation of his own statement in Bengalee, 'For two years I laboured under this disease, and scarcely slept for five months. On the 19th May,

I came to the Imambarah Hospital, and three or four persons tried to make me sleep, but all in vain. On the 3d June Dr. Esdaile having kindly undertaken my cure, with a great deal of labour, made me sleep, and took something out of my left cheek, which at that time I did not perceive. After the operation, I did not sleep for two nights, but after the third day, I have slept as usual.'[38]

Dr Esdaile was summoned to attend to the wife of Baboo Essanchunder Ghosaul (Ishan Chandra Ghoshal), a deputy magistrate of Hooghly on 6 June, at eight in the evening. Upon arrival, he found her in a state of severe convulsions, characterized by speechlessness, throat constriction, and intermittent rigidity and flexion of the body, reminiscent of tetanus and hydrophobia. The intensity of the convulsions rendered traditional medical interventions ineffective, as she was unable to breathe, let alone ingest medication. Dr Esdaile therefore employed his novel therapeutic approach, leveraging mesmerism to induce a state of catalepsy after nearly an hour of intense effort. As of 1 July, she has not experienced any recurrence of the convulsive episode, thereby attesting to the efficacy of this innovative treatment modality. Notably, a conjurer had been dispatched to provide relief, but arrived too late to be of assistance.[39] On 11 June Kaloo, a *fuqueer* (fakir), had an excrescence, larger than a man's fist. Dr Esdaile entranced him in a few minutes, on the first trial, and in the presence of Major Riddell, Captain Anderson, Mr Bennett, and Mr Jackson, dissected out the organ, but was obliged to sacrifice the glands, as it was a cartilaginous degeneration of all the structures of the part. The man did not awake till the amputation of the organ, after a long dissection.[40] A peasant, Toorab (thirty years old) presented with a chronic sinus tract, measuring six inches in length, located under the pectoral muscle, which had persisted for several months. On 16 June, despite various attempts, the lesion had resisted closure, necessitating surgical intervention. Under the induction of mesmerism by one of Dr Esdaile's assistants, the patient was rendered insensible, allowing for the successful excision of the diseased tract without his awareness. The patient was left in a sleeping state post-procedure. Upon awakening shortly thereafter, he expressed confusion regarding the origin of the blood, demonstrating minimal pain and no recollection of the surgical intervention performed while he was under mesmerism.[41]

The case of Oboychurn Roy (Abhay Charan Roy), a Hindu landowner, presented a remarkable instance of traumatic amputation, having suffered the loss of his left arm twelve days prior while defending his property against a group of bandits. Upon admission to the hospital on 10 July, physical examination revealed two distinct ligature-induced circular marks on his arm, a testament to the effective control of haemorrhaging. Notably, despite the high risk of gangrene, none had developed. Surgical intervention was necessary to remove several bone fragments, a procedure that typically elicits significant pain. However, following local and subsequently general mesmerism, the patient experienced considerable analgesia and promptly fell asleep within thirty minutes, achieving his first uninterrupted nocturnal rest since the traumatic event.[42]

The case of Napaul presented a complex and high-risk scenario that required a thorough and nuanced evaluation by Dr Esdaile. The subsequent analysis, presented below, provides a detailed explication of the multifaceted issues affecting Napaul, highlighting the severity and potential dangers inherent in this notable case study, as reported by Dr Esdaile. This case study offers a valuable opportunity for in-depth examination and analysis, shedding light on the intricacies and challenges posed by such exceptional circumstances.

> Aug. 23d. Napaul Bagdy, a husbandman, has a singular fungoid mass in the right groin; it is the size of a small cauliflower, and like it in appearance, the surface being whitish from sloughing. It spreads from a peduncle in the abdominal ring, and bleeds much when handled. His father says that, at his birth, there was only one testis in the scrotum, and no trace of the other was seen till he was six months old, when a swelling appeared in the groin. This gradually increased till his twelfth year, but was not painful or inconvenient. About this time he was attacked with fever, attended with increased sensibility and increase of size in the tumour, and the paroxysms came on twice a month, up to June last, when he applied to a barber-surgeon, who used means to ripen the

swelling. In the course of a few days it was punctured, and blood only followed. The opening was plugged as well as possible with a candle covered with cloth smeared with some ointment, but in a few days this came out, and the following day, a fungus shot out of the wound, and daily increased to its present size. It is now a very foul mass, its surface mortified, and the crevices filled with maggots. Aug. 26th.—He was mesmerised after two hours' trial, and the mass removed without his feeling it. Aug. 31st.—Discharged at his own request—wound looking well.[43]

On 1 September Raimgopal (Ram Gopal), a young Hindu, got a high syphilitic sore, about the size of half a lemon, on each side of his nates. He was entranced on the first trial; and in the presence of Dr James Clark Ross and Dr Charles T. Sissmore, Dr Esdaile turned him round like a log, and cut off both the excrescences level with the skin, then turned him back again, and left him sleeping. It is needless to say that he did not feel any pain during the operation.[44] On 18 September Morally Dass (Murli Das) a fifty-year-old peasant and Teg Ali Khan all suffering from different diseases were treated by this method. Gradually the experiment of mesmeric anaesthesia became popular among the people. Students and doctors gathered in the Imambarah Hospital to learn more about the method.[45]

A series of surgical interventions were performed by Dr James Esdaile, utilizing mesmerism as an anaesthetic agent, and witnessed by various esteemed observers, including Mr Sutherland, Dr Owen, Reverend Mr Bradbury, Major

Riddle, Mr Higgen, Mr Muller, Mr Graves, Messrs. Savigny, Mr Calder, Mr Bartlett, Mr Russell, Judge of Hooghly, Major Smitt, H.M. Dr Scott, Captain Smythe, Captain D.L. Richardson, and Mr Samuells, Burdwan collector. The patients who underwent these procedures included Nazir (8 and 10 October), who suffered from an enlarged and scirrhous testis and underwent extirpation; Gooroochuan Shah (Guru Charan Saha; 24 October), who had a monstrous tumour resected; Ameer Mullick (16 November), who underwent tumour resection for a large tumour; Bungsee (Bangshi; 18 November), who had a twenty-eight-pound tumour removed; Mahesh Banerjee (26 November), who underwent surgical correction of an enlarged testis and scrotal hernia; and Jano (Jana; 14 and 15 December), a blind prisoner who was mesmerised in preparation for potential surgical intervention to address cataracts in both eyes.[46]

The aforementioned cases serve merely as illustrative examples of exceptional instances, whereas James Esdaile's seminal work *Mesmerism in Colonial India* provides a comprehensive and in-depth examination of each case study, offering a rich and nuanced exploration of the subject matter. For a detailed and erudite analysis of these cases, Esdaile's book is an indispensable resource, providing scholars with a definitive and authoritative reference.

After gaining confidence in its ultimate success, on 22 January 1846 Dr Esdaile submitted a detailed list of seventy-three mesmeric anaesthetic surgical operations[47] of the last eight months.

Mesmeric Anaesthetic Surgeries at the Calcutta Mesmeric Hospital

Report of A Return Showing The Number Of Painless Surgical Operations Performed At Hooghly, During The Last Eight Months.	
Arm amputated	1
Breast ditto	1
Tumour extracted from the upper jaw	1
Scirrhus testium extirpated	2
Penis amputated	2
Contracted knees straightened	3
Ditto arms	3
Operations for cataract	3
Large tumour in the groin cut off	1
Operations for Hydrocele	7
Ditto Dropsy	2
Actual Cautery applied to a sore	1
Muriatic acid ditto	2
Unhealthy sores pared down	7
Abscesses opened	5
Sinus, six inches long, laid open	1
	1
Heel flayed	1
End of thumb cut off	3
Teeth extracted	1
Gum cut away Prepuce cut off	3
Piles ditto	1
Great toe nails cut out by the roots	5
Seton introduced from ankle to knee	1
Large tumour on leg removed	1
Scrotal tumours, weighing from 8 lb. to 80 lb., removed 17, painless	14
Total Operations	73

He also sent a report to *The Englishman*,

> To the Editor of the Englishman.
> Sir - Before proceeding to join the army, I have the pleasure to send you a 'resume' of my mesmeric practice during the last eight months. My experience has demonstrated the singular and beneficial influence exerted by Mesmerism over the constitution of the Natives of Bengal, and that painless surgical operations, with other advantages, are their natural birthright, of which they will no longer be deprived, I hope. Duty calls me to another and more extensive field, where I hope to work out this curious and interesting subject in all its practical details, and to ascertain to what extent other varieties of mankind are capable of being benefitted by this natural curative power.
> I am, your obedient servant,
> James Esdaile, M. D.
> Hooghly, 22d Jan., 1846

Dr Esdaile suggested that mesmeric anaesthesia should be practised in all the Indian hospitals. With this intention he wrote a letter to Dr Elliotson,

> Dear Sir.-In consequence of the late unexpected engagements with the Sikhs, 3000 wounded have been thrown on our hands, without any provision being made to receive them, and the civil surgeons are therefore ordered to join the army, by post, with the least possible delay. I

start tomorrow, but before going, cannot deny myself the pleasure of informing you of the establishment of mesmerism in Bengal, I may say, in India. I may claim the undivided credit of having introduced this great blessing into India, and of having demonstrated the wonderful extent to which the natives of this country can be benefitted by it. But here, and elsewhere, the principal honour will justly revert to you, for without your courageous and independent advocacy of the truth, the different nations of the earth would have been deprived of this most valuable natural remedy for an indefinite length of time.

I leave a Mesmeric Corps here, paid by the Government, so that the good done will not be undone by my departure. I hope soon to establish Mesmerism in the other extremity of Hindostan, and to benefit even our enemies by it. Permit me to congratulate you on the happy results of your labours, which will be an encouragement to others not to be ashamed of the truth.

I have the pleasure to enclose you my seventy-fourth painless operation, and send you by this mail, a newspaper containing a summary of my mesmeric doings for the last eight months. I have also sent the MS. of a work, called "Mesmerism in India," to my friends by this mail, and if it finds a publisher, you will find curious matter in it.

I am, with much respect,
Yours truly,
JAMES ESDAILE, M.D.,
Civil Surgeon.[48]

Dr Esdaile executed a total of seventy-three surgical procedures devoid of pain between April 1845 and January 1846, notwithstanding the lack of governmental support. He subsequently continued his practice, performing an additional twenty-nine operations at Hooghly Charity and Jail Hospital from January to July 1846. These original case reports were disseminated through esteemed newspapers and medical journals, and subsequently compiled in *The Zoist* under the editorship of Dr Elliotson. The following section presents a paraphrased collection of the most remarkable cases from this mesmeric surgical series.

One notable case from this series occurred on 28 January 1846, when Jabour Dhun Shah underwent the excision of a forty-pound scrotal tumour while in a mesmeric trance, without experiencing any pain. This operation was witnessed by Commissioner of Police Mr S. Wanchope, who attested to the patient's insensibility during surgery and provided the following certificate:

> Certificate, That I witnessed the above operation, and that the man on awaking declared to me, that he not only felt no pain during or after the operation, but was now in perfect health and strength, and as a proof, rose from the bed on which he had been operated upon, and walked to another with the most perfect ease, refusing all assistance.

Furthermore, Jabour Dhun Shah dictated a letter to his father through a friend, which was translated as follows:

Your servant, Jabour Dhun Shah, bowing respectfully, begs to inform you, that through your blessing, I arrived at Hooghly on the evening of the 26th Jan. On my going to the hospital next day, I saw the native sub-assistant surgeon (the Doctor Sahib not being present) who put me to sleep, and then examined my disease. This morning, the 28th Jan., I was put to sleep at 10 o'clock, a.m., and the tumour was cut off without my feeling any pain. Being then asleep, I know nothing that was done. I awoke in an hour after, and saw the tumour lying on the ground. The Sahibs questioned me, and I answered quite comfortably, without any pain about me. You need not be anxious about me, I will often communicate to you the state of my health. Hooghly Hospital, 28th Jan., 1846.[49]

These accounts demonstrate the efficacy of mesmerism in surgical procedures, as evident in the successful operation performed on Jabour Dhun Shah.

Under the observation of esteemed medical professionals, including Dr Clapperton and Sub-assistant surgeon Budan Chunder Chowdary, Dr James Esdaile executed surgical interventions leveraging mesmerism as an anaesthetic modality. Modoo (Madhu; 8 February) presented with a fistulous sore in the right cheek, while Ramdhun (12 February), a forty-year-old male, exhibited phimosis. Guru Charan (Gour Charan; 18 February), a prisoner, displayed a fistulous opening in the chin, and

Rasso (21 February), a fifty-six-year-old Hindu female, suffered from rheumatism. Additionally, Ruttun (Ratan; 4 March), an eighty-year-old male, presented with Ischuria vesicles, and Puddo (Padma; 5 March), a thirty-two-year-old husbandman, experienced rheumatic pain in the elbow and ankle. Further cases included Solim (Selim; 7 March), a forty-year-old Muslim male with severe pain in his right shoulder, and Shaikh Golam (22 February), a prisoner afflicted with rheumatism. The cohort also comprised Gungaram Doss (Ganga Ram Das; 6 April), a fifteen-year-old beggar with deep extensive sores, and Newfar Bagdy (Nefear Bagchi; 6 April), a thirty-four-year-old *coolie* with a compound fracture in both bones of the right leg. Moreover, Kashi Nath Roy (8 April), a thirty-five-year-old male, presented with a scrotum tumour, Ramdhun Ghose (8 April), a forty-year-old cow keeper, exhibited a disease in the right ear and a fistulous sore behind it, and Bagoban Doss (Bhagwan Das; 8 April), a fifty-five-year-old sirdar bearer, displayed a large thirty pounds scrotal tumour.[50]

Now, after the completion of 102 painless surgeries through mesmeric trance, Dr Esdaile had to directly communicate to the deputy governor of Bengal.[51] During that time Sir Herbert Madock was the deputy governor of Bengal.[52] On 31 July 1846 the deputy governor was ordered to form a mesmeric committee with seven delegated members to monitor the mesmerising painless surgery performed by Esdaile and collect reports from the same. The seven members of this committee were: J. Atkinson, Esq. Inspector General of Hospital and Chairman of The Committee, E.M. Gordon, Esq., J.J. Jackson, Esq., Surgeon, Native Hospital, D. Stewart, Esq., M.D. Presidency Surgeon, W.B. O' Shaughnessy, Esq., M.D. Secretary of The Committee, James Hume, Esq., A Rogers Esq.

On 9 October 1846, the committee submitted a detailed report based on the experiment of ten surgical operations under mesmeric anaesthesia. The report was submitted to the Secretary of the Government of Bengal.

Fourteen meetings had been held from 7:30 am to 10 am from 7 to 19 September in the presence of seven members and Dr Esdaile. On 7 September 1846, a meeting was held at the Hooghly Native Hospital. The President was Dr Atkinson, and other members were Dr J. Jackson, Dr W.B. O'Shaughnessy, E.M. Gordon, A. Rogers, and J.A.S. Hume. Dr W.B. O'Shaughnessy was directed to act as secretary and recorded each day's proceedings, also keeping the minutes of the cases. All the records were explained in the next meeting in front of Dr Esdaile. On the following page is the complete list of patients subjected to Dr Esdaile's mesmeric experiment under the invigilation of the mesmeric committee.[53]

No.	Name	Age	Admitted	Disease	Duration	Operation
1	Cheedam (Chidam)	40	7th September	Double Hydrocele	Several Months	Apparently painless.
2	Bissonath (Biswanath)	20	7th September	Tumour of Scrotum	Same	Out
3	Nilmoney Dutt	45	7th September	Same	Same	Apparently painless.
4	Neelchul (Nilachal)	35	7th September	Phymosis	Same	Out
5	Deeloo (Dilu)	40	7th September	Double Hydrocele	3 Years	Out
6	Jahiroodeen (Jahiruddin)	33	7th September	Penis Hypertrophy	2 Years	Doubtful
7	Dohmun	40	10th September	Hyper of Scrotum	Several Months	Doubtful
8	Ramchund (Ram Chand)	18	13th September	Hyper of Scrotum	2 Years	Doubtful
9	Hyder Khan	30	16th September	Leg Mortification	15 Days	Apparently painless.
10	Murli Doss (Murli Das)	30	14th September	Hyper of Scrotum	6 Years	Apparently painless.

Not all of the above-mentioned patients were mesmerised. Three cases out of the ten, Bissonath, Deeloo, and Neelchul, were dismissed without satisfactory effect; Bisonath suffered from a slight cough to which Dr Esdaile considered rendering the mesmeric manipulation ineffectual; Deeloo on the fifth day for having taken spirits, and Neelchul (Nilachal) having resisted the mesmeric processes during eleven days without conclusive result. In seven cases, in a period varying from one to seven sittings, deep sleep followed the performance of the processes described above. In its most perfect state, this sleep differed from ordinary natural sleep. For instance, loud noises could not arouse the individual and the pupils were insensible to light. In some cases, apparently perfect insensibility to pain was witnessed in burning, pinching, and cutting the skin and other sensitive organs. In seven cases, surgical operations were performed in the state of sleep described above among them; in the case of Nilmoney Dutt, there was not the slightest indication of the operation having been felt by the patient. It consisted of the removal of a tumour. It lasted four minutes. The patient's hands or legs were not held. He did not move or groan nor did his countenance change. In another case, Hyder Khan, an emaciated man, was suffering from mortification of the leg. An amputation of the thigh was performed, which showed no sign of causing pain. In a third case, Murli Doss (Murli Das), a palanquin bearer from Hooghly, was admitted with considerable hypertrophy of the scrotum. The operation he underwent was very severe, because he moved his body and arms, breathing in gasps, but his countenance underwent little change, and the features expressed no suffering, and on awaking, he declared he knew of nothing having been done to him during his sleep. However, in the case of Ramchund (Ram Chand) two separate incisions were operated; just as the first was completed in about four minutes, his body started writhing and he woke up with distortion on his face. On proceeding to the second step, he shouted aloud in pain and terror and protested so violently that the operator had to stop. On 9 October 1946, Hurronundo Saha (Harananda Saha), aged twenty-seven, hearing that Dr Esdaile was in

Calcutta, came to the Native Hospital with an enormous scrotal tumour. It measured seven feet in circumference and two feet round its neck. Dr Esdaile operated the 103 lbs tumour in the presence of Dr Duncan Stewart, the Presidency Surgeon.[54]

On 9 October 1846 two of the committee members James Atkinson and W.B. O'Shaughnessy submitted their final report to F.J. Halliday.[55] They reported that the seven cases of mesmeric operation in which deep sleep was produced were in all appearance, perfectly painless. The patients expressed no knowledge or recollection of what had occurred, complained of no pain, till their attention was directed to the place where the operation had been performed. They attributed great merit to Dr Esdaile for the zeal, ability and boldness with which he had taken up the challenge and also remarked that his sphere of work had been limited. They hoped that his further investigations may be extended to European as well as native patients.

Healing Reimagined: The Birth of Calcutta Mesmeric Hospital (1846 to 1848)

On the basis of the above positive report given by the Mesmeric Committee it was hoped their inquiries would prove the efficacy of using mesmerism and that they would be able to induce the government to introduce its practice into general hospitals. The Mesmeric Committee had met fourteen times, each sitting being of two hours duration, attending to the different cases. Upon receiving a favourable report, the then Governor of Bengal issued an order to open an experimental mesmeric hospital near Motts Lane, Calcutta in November 1846:

> With this view His Honor has determined, with the sanction of the Supreme Government, to place Dr. Esdaile for one year in charge of a small experimental hospital in some favorable situation in Calcutta, in order that he may, as recommended by the Committee, extend his investigations to the applicability of this alleged agency to all descriptions of cases, Medical as well as Surgical, and all classes of patients, European as well as Native. Dr. Esdaile will be directed to encourage the resort to his hospital of all respectable persons desirous of satisfying themselves of the nature and the effect of his experiments, especially Medical and Scientific individuals in or out of the Service; and His Honor will nominate from among the Medical Officers of the Presidency, "Visitors", Whose duty it will be to visit the hospital from time to time, inspect Dr. Esdaile's proceedings, without exercising any interference, and occasionally, or when called on, report upon them, through the Medical Board, for the information of Government. On these Reports will mainly depend what further steps the Government may deem it expedient to take in the matter.[56]

After the establishment of the Calcutta Mesmeric Hospital, several newspapers and magazines wrote about it. At this time, the *Bengal Hurkaru* opined that the government was determined on giving Dr J. Esdaile a much wider theatre for the demonstration of his experiments.[57] Meanwhile *The Englishman*, a popular newspaper, commented that they are glad to observe that Dr Esdaile satisfied the government committee, and that he was immediately appointed as the head of a Mesmeric Hospital.[58] The *Ceylon Observer*, pointed out that the new hospital would be advantageous for mesmerism as it was a remedial agent which could be applied to a wide variety of cases, which did not fall into the hands of the surgeon, and though the effects on these were less striking than in such terrible operations as those which were recorded, yet they were not less important; and considering the great advantages possessed by a public institution, one could scarcely doubt that the foundation of the intended hospital would prove an era in the medical annals of India.[59] *The Calcutta Star* concurred with committee member Mr James Hume in his objections to certain paragraphs which were calculated to create an unfavourable impression of mesmerism as a surgical and medical agent, neither warranted by what was seen, nor by the reasoning applied to what was not seen. *The Friend of India* spoke of the evident reluctance that the members of the committee, with one exception, had manifested in admitting the facts established by these experiments. The deputy governor wished all classes of the community to benefit from this institution, and said that rooms would be set apart for wealthy persons to be mesmerised so that all classes of the society could enjoy painless surgery. The Calcutta Mesmeric Hospital was built experimentally for a total of eighteen months.[60]

Chronicles of Mesmeric Surgery: Tales from Calcutta's Healing Haven

Since the establishment of the Calcutta Mesmeric Hospital, the successful treatment of patients over the eighteen-month period has been classified into two distinct categories based on the complexity and significance of the ailments addressed. The first category comprises treatments for patients suffering from complex and severe diseases, while the second encompasses more common and general ailments. These two sections illustrate the range of illnesses successfully treated through mesmerism, accompanied by basic patient information. Amid the multitude of cases managed at the hospital, a select few, characterized by their complexity and clinical significance, merit particular attention. The following section provides a paraphrased account of such noteworthy cases.

On the wintry day of 3 December 1846, Baboo Nundkishore Roy (Nanda Kishore Roy) the diligent bookkeeper of Messrs. Lattey, Brothers and Co. of Kolkata, walked through the hospital's doors carrying a burden that matched his apprehension. Adorning his person was a conspicuous tumour, an unwelcome growth rivalling the proportions of a grown man's cranium. The date etched into history as 6 February 1847 saw the convergence of medical minds – Dr J. Esdaile was joined by the astute presence of Dr Thompson,

Dr Mouat, and the notable Mr R. O'Shaughnessy. As curious onlookers, they observed as skilled hands sought to reclaim normalcy for Baboo Nundkishore Roy. A mesmerising procedure unfolded, bearing the promise of relief, and the world watched with bated breath.[61]

In another corner of the hospital's chronicles, the narrative interweaved with the story of Monoo, a thirty-five-year-old man who traversed a formidable 200-mile journey from Cuttack. Whispers of a miraculous operation, unaccompanied by pain, had reached Monoo's ears, guiding him to the doors of the hospital. A modest tumour, concealed upon his frame, was not to be the master of his fate. The Nabab of Murshidabad, along with the esteemed Mr Torrens and Dr Grant, lent their presence to the occasion. The tapestry of events unfurled on 9 January 1847, as the mesmerising trance of science commenced. Mesmerised Monoo, shielded from pain's cruel embrace, bore witness to the unveiling of his affliction – a hydrocele resting on his left flank. The surgical symphony orchestrated on 14 February 1847, culminated in the liberation of pent-up fluids, and Monoo awoke from his mesmerised slumber with gratitude for an undisturbed repose.[62]

Amidst the mosaic of patients, the story of Bhoyrub Doss, known to some as Bhairab Das, was etched with fortitude. Dwelling in the confines of Dingavanga, Kolkata, Bhoyrub Doss bore a cross of sixteen long years – a tumour, unbidden and persistent, stretched its dominion, challenging his resolve. 20 March 1847, stood as a defining moment, an intersection of fate and medical mastery. Dr Esdaile, his hands guided by expertise and aided by a congregation of inquisitive gazes – both native and European – faced the task. The theatre of operation saw the successful wresting of a colossal tumour, a burden weighing fifteen pounds, from Bhoyrub Doss's frame.[63]

The Calcutta Mesmeric Hospital, with its roster of remarkable cases, each imbued with a distinctive narrative, encapsulated a slice of medical history where mesmerism intertwined with surgical advancement. The stories of Nundkishore Roy, Monoo and Bhoyrub Doss stood as beacons, illuminating the path towards medical exploration, pioneering the limits of human intervention, and offering respite from afflictions that once held sway over the lives of the afflicted.

Amidst the corridors of the Calcutta Mesmeric Hospital, a series of extraordinary cases painted a vivid tableau of medical marvels. On 20 March 1847, Huro (Haru), a twenty-five-year-old peasant woman from Chinsurah of Hooghly, entered the annals of history with her plight. For two long years, cartilaginous tumours had clung tenaciously to the upper regions of each ear, a burden she carried with quiet determination. As the clock struck twelve on 31 March, a gathering of Europeans and natives bore witness to a remarkable feat. With deliberate precision, the skilled hands of medical practitioners embarked on a delicate trance of dissection. The ethereal realm of mesmerism cocooned Huro, her body a portrait of tranquility, even as the tumours met their end. A mere ten minutes post-operation, she roused from her mesmeric slumber, her reflection in a looking glass unveiled the transformation that had transpired. The painless passage from unconsciousness to consciousness left her marvelling, the memory of the procedure elusive until half an hour had whispered its passage.[64] In the wake of Huro's tale, the chronicle shifted to Sonatun Mahetie, a weathered labourer of thirty-two years. He had journeyed from the far reaches of Bhadrak, Cuttack, a fourteen-day odyssey to find solace. The baggage he carried, both literal and metaphorical, was profound. An eighteen-year-long companionship with a cartilaginous scrotal tumour had been etched upon him, a burden surpassed only by his ailing leg, afflicted by the cruel grip of elephantiasis. The size of the tumour, formidable and unyielding, defied expectations, its sixteen-pound weight a testament to its dominance. The stage was set, and the date aligned, as 31 March 1847 ushered in the transformation. A mesmerised trance enveloped Sonatun Mahetie, his journey through the realm of unconsciousness preserving the sanctity of the procedure. Dr Esdaile, orchestrating the delicate ballet of surgery, found his patient's mesmeric slumber unbroken, a testament to the power of the mind's embrace.[65] In the tapestry of the hospital's endeavours, Shaik Koochill emerged, a fifty-year-old cart driver hailing from Karawa, a corner of the 24-Pergunnahs. His existence had been shadowed by a hypertrophic scrotal tumour, an eight-year companion that had worn his spirit.

The journey towards relief commenced on 1 April 1847, culminating in a harmonious interplay of mesmeric trance and surgical prowess on 10 April. A ten-pound weight was cast aside with surgical precision, and Shaik Koochill lay, an inert figure, a tableau of tranquility rarely witnessed. It was a half-hour symphony of stillness, a lifeless reprieve that gave way only when the hands of the surgeon shifted their focus. From the realm of the unconscious, Shaik Koochill emerged, his consciousness unmarred by the passage of surgical mastery.[66]

The saga, with its twists and turns, took a final turn on 4 April 1847, as Bonmallee Bhuttacharge (Banamali Bhattacharya), a Brahmin of twenty-six years, entered the fray. His abode in Sookchur of the 24-Pergunnahs concealed a secret, a scrotal tumour of immense proportions, a burden that had lingered for nine long years. Battling periodic fever, he embarked on a journey to reclaim his vitality. The 22nd of April marked a pivotal moment as the weighty tumour, tipping the scales at thirty pounds, met its end. The operation, a carefully choreographed act, unfolded to the rhythm of mesmerism's embrace. As the mass yielded to the surgeon's touch, Bonmallee Bhuttacharge's tranquility held firm. A momentary shift, an unintelligible cry, marked the crescendo of the operation, yet even this ephemeral disturbance was swiftly quelled. A clean sheet draped him, obscured the traces of the surgical ballet, and his slumber remained unbroken. The realm of pain eluded him, a testament to the power of mesmerism's touch.[67] The Calcutta

Mesmeric Hospital, a stage for medical marvels, saw its halls graced by stories of courage and transformation.

From Huro's quiet awakening to Sonatun Mahetie's steadfast journey, Shaik Koochill's serene reprieve, and Bonmallee Bhuttacharge's dreamless slumber, each chapter carved its mark in the annals of surgical history, all under the mesmerising embrace of medical exploration.

On 10 May 1847, Gopaul Doss (Gopal Das), a robust bearer of forty years, traversed a considerable distance from Ballessur (Balasore) to seek solace. His frame, large and muscular, carried a burden that had plagued him for five years – a small yet persistent hypertrophic scrotal tumour. The stage was set on 12 May, as the luminous presence of Mr Halliday, Major Sage, Mr Simms, Mr Fraser, and Dr Jackson bore witness to the transformative act. Dr Esdaile, the orchestrator of mesmerism's touch, guided the surgical journey that liberated Gopaul Doss from his burden. The weighty tumour, a ten-pound reminder of his suffering, met its end under the skilled hands of the mesmeric surgeon. The aftermath revealed an intriguing facet of the patient's experience by Bengali scholar Mr Kemp – Gopaul Doss, once roused from his mesmeric slumber, reluctantly recounted his operation encounter, his desire to return to slumber a testament to the comfort found within.[68]

A young East Indian named Miss Gordon stepped into the hospital's embrace on 23 December 1847. A tale of two years marred by the enlargement of throat and neck glands unfolded before the mesmeric practitioners.

The disfigurement, profound in its extent, could only be comprehended through visual representation. Yet, with the mesmeric blade, a painless extraction of the afflicted glands transpired. In this delicate act, the hospital's narrative expanded to encompass Europeans, as they too became beneficiaries of the mesmeric touch.[69] The 15th of January marked Mr Des Bruslais a French merchantman's arrival, his existence shackled by six months of chronic rheumatism and the cruel grip of an enlarged, tender, and stiff left elbow. The mesmeric process unfurled its enigmatic tapestry, as Mr Des Bruslais succumbed to its embrace for three-quarters of a day. Upon emerging from the mesmeric trance, the pain that once held dominion over his elbow had been banished, replaced by a newfound sense of well-being.[70]

The 18th of February ushered in the presence of Sarah Goodall, a mere eleven years of age. For eight years, the periodic onslaught of inflammation in neck and ear glands had marred her youthful days. A symphony of mesmeric influences played out as, by the 22nd, the tenderness and swelling of her afflicted glands yielded to the touch, a testament to the mesmeric healing that had unfolded.[71]

Amidst the hospital's corridors, Shaik Ameerresidedin (Amir Sad Uddin), a fifty-year-old resident of Calcutta, grappled with a stiff ankle that had held him captive for five years. The joint's pain, swelling, and immobility gave way to a mesmeric miracle. On 15 February, a transformed Shaik Ameerresidedin walked with newfound grace, pain relegated to the past, a once-swollen ankle now restored.[72] Frances

Ann Elliot's tale unveiled itself on 21 January 1847. Chronic rheumatism had woven its threads through her life, birthed enlarged glands and burs on the inner side of her right ankle. A tangible presence, akin to a hen's egg, burdened her. The 23rd of April marked a turning point, as the ulcer's healing was accompanied by the departure of swelling and pain. The mesmeric blade had sculpted a path to liberation, enabled her to traverse the distance from hospital to home without hindrance, a testament to the mesmeric touch's efficacy.[73]

Within these narratives, the Calcutta Mesmeric Hospital's legacy thrived, each account illuminating the profound impact of mesmerism on affliction, pain and healing. In the gentle embrace of mesmeric trance, a symphony of transformation played out, paving the way for a future shaped by the fusion of science and mesmeric exploration. On 7 April 1847, the hospital's corridors welcomed Bhoobunmohun Dey (Bhuban Mohan Dey), a peddler from Calcutta, his life tainted by hemiplegia's cruel grasp for sixteen days. His left side bore the weight of complete palsy, his visage marked by a permanent distortion. Yet, on 21 April, the stage was set for a mesmeric marvel. Through surgical mastery, the rigidity that held his left side captive yielded, the once clenched fist unfurled, the facial distortion softened, and the left leg regained its mobility. The mesmeric touch, guided by Dr Esdaile's expertise, had breathed life into his paralysis.[74] The narrative then turned to Jhung Nathea, a ten-year-old whose journey into mesmerism began with a perplexing malady. The dawn of 18 December 1847 saw his left arm rendered powerless overnight. A mesmeric intervention on the same day marked the start of a miraculous journey. By the 22nd, his strength returned, and as December drew to a close, Jhung Nathea emerged, movement restored to his left arm.

24 May 1847 marked Muneeroodeen's presence, a labourer of thirty years tethered to a scrotal tumour's weight and the grasp of elephantiasis. The electromagnetic machine's embrace brought forth convulsive movements, rendering him passive as a corpse. De-mesmerisation brought partial awakening, a plea for sleep replacing the cacophony of movements. Mesmerism also worked in the lunatic asylum, in this regard Dr Esdaile's mesmeric treatment had been published in *The Calcutta Medical Journal* on the treated eight case reports.[75]

Madhu, professionally known as Madhu mallee, entered the narrative on 8 June 1847. A small scrotal tumour marred his existence for three years. Dr Palmer bore witness as the operation, a mirror of previous cases, unfolded before their eyes. Perfect insensibility marked each step, a testament to mesmerism's profound embrace.[76] In the hallowed halls of the Calcutta Mesmeric Hospital, the journey through mesmerism's touch unfurled, stories of transformation marked by pain's retreat, paralysis's release, and burdens lifted. Each patient, a testament to the uncharted territories of mesmeric exploration, carved their mark within the history of medical science.

On 7 July 1847, the hospital's embrace enveloped Moteewoolla Jemadar, a fifty-year-old resident of

Alelompore in Zillah Burdwan. Eight years of burden had been shouldered, the weight of a moderate-sized scrotal tumour shaping his existence. Midnight on 13 July brought forth a symphony of surgery, a relentless battle against the mass's hardness and the testes' hidden depths. Dr Esdaile's skilled hands navigated the intricate trance, leaving no part untamed. The tumour's weight, a staggering twenty pounds, rested separate from its host. Moteewoolla Jemadar stirred, his slumber yielding to consciousness, and a newfound sensation of smarting greeted his awakening. The reality of his transformation unfolded as the severed mass was unveiled before him. His gratitude poured forth, blessing Dr Esdaile with visions of golden palanquins and carriages, a testament to the profound impact of mesmeric healing.[77]

The 28th of October 1847 witnessed the arrival of Shaikh Armon, a shopkeeper of twenty years from Khalasitollah in Kolkata. Lumbago had tethered his nights to pain's embrace, his limp a constant reminder of his affliction. Mesmeric intervention unfurled a different path. As the 4th of November embraced the night, Shaikh Armon slept within the cocoon of mesmeric trance, his pain yielding to restful slumber. The 7th of November revealed a transformed soul, unburdened by pain, liberated from the confines of a limp, and restored to the rhythm of daily life.[78]

Chunga Singh, a thirty-year-old labourer dwelling in Bura Bajar (Barabazar) of Calcutta, grappled with acute rheumatism's torment. The articulations that defined motion had surrendered to swelling and pain. Dr Esdaile's mesmeric touch became the healer's wand, evoking change without the need for surgical steel. Three times a day, the mesmerist's art unfolded, and within the embrace of mesmeric trance, Chunga Singh embarked on a journey toward liberation. Gradual steps paved the way, a night of restlessness eventually giving way to profound slumber. The 31st of December unveiled a transformed soul, now able to run and jump with abandon, a testament to mesmeric healing's potency.[79] Within the walls of the Calcutta Mesmeric Hospital, these tales of healing unfurled, each account a testament to the power of mesmeric intervention. From Moteewoolla Jemadar's late-night surgery to Shaikh Armon's restful slumber, and Chunga Singh's steady path to recovery, the hospital's legacy stood as a beacon of hope and transformation.

Notably, not only were major cases treated successfully through mesmerism, the process also yielded favourable results in intriguing and fascinating instances. Chand Khan, one of the individuals who had undergone experimental procedures in the previous month to study the effects of cold on mesmeric sleep, had his tumour meticulously examined on 1 January. Moving to 2 April, Bhugeeruth (Bhagirath), a thirty-two-year-old husbandman, arrived at the residence of Dr James Esdaile in the morning. He presented symptoms indicative of a stone condition that had been afflicting him for a span of two years. Over the course of the last year, his agony had been unrelenting, and he experienced considerable discomfort even while walking.[80] On 6 April 1847, a surgical operation was conducted on Bhugeeruth in relation to his ailment. An intriguing aspect emerged during the procedure when, as the stone was traversing his pelvis, he opened his eyes and appeared to possess his senses. However, upon the operation's completion, he recollected only a sensation of something yielding within his abdomen, followed by a warmth emanating from the wound site. Echoing previous instances, his visual acuity remained impaired for a period subsequent to his eye-opening, and the first distinct sight he beheld was that of the stone, presented before him. It was at this juncture that he became conscious of the presence of the gentlemen surrounding him. The weight of the removed stone was measured at twenty grains.[81]

Advancing to 14 April, Shaik Morad, a forty-year-old tailor residing in Sobhabazar, Calcutta, exhibited a scrotal tumour that had persisted for six years. On 26 April, an operation was performed on him by Esdaile. Notably, Shaik Morad had been disturbed prior to the procedure and regained awareness only after being draped with a clean sheet. Strikingly, he remained oblivious to the surgical intervention that had transpired. While he acknowledged the customary sensation of weight, he reported an absence of pain.[82] The narrative expands to 4 May 1847, when Myzoodeen (Maijuddin), a twenty-five-year-old Khidmutgar in the service of Mr Lindstedt, residing in Kalitollah, Hooghly, presented a small scrotal tumour of two years' duration. Coinciding with lunar phase changes, the tumour would manifest alongside episodes of fever, occurring twice each month. The ensuing operation on 9 April unfolded in a manner consistent with previous cases, characterized by the absence of sensibility during the procedure.[83]

The account also encompasses the instance of Wullee Mahmood (Wali Muhammad), a thirty-year-old boatman from Chittagong (Chattogram). Admitted on 14 January 1847, he had been grappling with rheumatism for a duration of five years. Subsequent to mesmerisation on 25 January 1847, he underwent a remarkable transformation, reporting an absence of ankle pain and newfound capabilities to walk, run, and jump without experiencing discomfort.[84]

In a sequence of diverse instances, the impact of mesmerism on varied medical conditions comes to light. Firstly, we encounter Mr Johnson, a thirty-four-year-old European gentleman, who suffered a severe fever three years earlier. Subsequently, he battled persistent nervous headaches that initially occurred daily for eight months and then assumed an irregular pattern. It was only after undergoing mesmerism that he found respite, having previously found little relief through conventional medical interventions.[85] As 5 April 1847 arrives, Beeja, a thirty-year-old Syce residing in Calcutta, emerges into focus. He had endured a bothersome stiffened arm for about six months, accompanied by significant pain and swelling. A remarkable transformation took place by 30 April, wherein both pain and swelling receded. Beeja regained considerable range of motion, exemplified by his ability to stretch and bend his arm with renewed ease. Notably, the bursa enlargement remained unchanged. By 19 May, the arm's restoration was pronounced, and Beeja declared a full recovery in its utilization.[86]

The narrative shifts to Nobin, a thirty-year-old labourer from Joypore in Cuttack, who was transferred to the Mesmeric Hospital on 4 April due to persistent epilepsy spanning two years. Employing the technique of mesmeric trance, efforts were made to address his condition.[87] Subsequently, on 29 May 1847, Gobind Chunder (Gobinda Chandra), a thirty-two-year-old beggar from Ramkistopore (Ramkrishnapur), takes centre stage. For eight long years, he endured the burden of a scrotal tumour. On 4 June, a surgical procedure was conducted, notable for Gobind Chunder's complete immobility and apparent lack of awareness during the operation. Astonishingly, he awoke naturally fifteen minutes post-operation, displaying no recognition of the surgical intervention that had taken place.[88]

As the narrative unfolds to 10 July 1847, Shamchunder Dutt (Shyamchundra Dutta), a forty-year-old shopkeeper residing in the village of Zingrapolasee in Hooghly, emerges with a longstanding struggle against hypertrophied scrotum and scirrhous testes, a plight spanning six years. The surgical procedure was executed on 12 July while he remained insensible, though a slight movement and muted sounds marked the procedure's conclusion. Consistent application of mesmerism was ensured until all vascular connections were secured. The patient regained consciousness approximately forty-five minutes after the operation, noting irritation at the operated site. Though he reported a slight sense of weakness, his sleep remained undisturbed, devoid of dreams.[89]

Bideadhur (Bidya Dhar), a sixteen-year-old labourer from Budruck in the Cuttack district came to the Calcutta Mesmeric Hospital on 12 July 1847. He suffered a grievous injury to his left great toe, crushed in an accident involving a substantial country boat two months prior. The wound deteriorated, prompting the removal of the affected portion up to the second joint on 14 July. Remarkably, after the procedure, Bideadhur remained in a deep slumber for roughly half an hour, awakening to acknowledge that the pain had notably subsided in comparison to pre-sleep sensations. This serves as a striking illustration of mesmerism's ability to alleviate acute pain.[90]

On 1 August 1847, Seetaram (Sitaram), a fifty-year-old porter residing in Kelore, Cuttack, encountered a small scrotal tumour that had persisted for a lengthy twenty-two years. Intervention on 7 August yielded a passive response, akin to a lifeless state, from the patient. A slight movement was observed in his left leg when the arteries were being secured. Roughly an hour and a half after the procedure, the patient awoke, reporting a lack of weakness and a smarting sensation at the operated site, unaware that the tumour had been excised.[91]

On 17 June 1847 Buddun chunder Kowr (Budhan Chandra Kewra), aged fifty, a letter receiver in the General Post Office residing at Entallee, Kolkata, had been troubled with a scrotal tumour for eleven years. On 3 October, in the presence of Dr Mouat his forty-pound tumour was operated.[92] On 22 October 1847, Susteedoss (Shashti Das), a labourer aged thirty-five, native of Angoona, in the Burdwan district, had a small scrotal tumour for six years. He was operated on 25 October. During the operation, he remained motionless and quiet, except towards the end, when he gently turned his face from one side to the other, and his countenance convulsed. However, he did not open his eyes or moan.[93]

A noteworthy instance transpired on 7 November 1847, involving Gopeedoss Sirdar (Gopi Das Sardar), a bearer hailing from Durmanugur, district Balessur. Having experienced a small scrotal tumour for five years, he was directed to the Calcutta Mesmeric Hospital by his friend Bhugwandoss (Bhagwan Das) who had undergone a similar procedure under Dr Esdaile's care in Hooghly the previous year.[94]

Shifting to 23 October 1847, Horry (Hori), a water carrier of thirty years, was besieged by a small scrotal tumour persisting over a five-year duration. Hailing from Cuttack, they journeyed with the aspiration of a painless removal. On 2 November, Dr James Esdaile performed the operation.[95]

Similarly, Chundechurn (Chandi Charan), a forty-two-year-old pleader affiliated with the Sudder Ameen's Court in Sylhet, bore a considerable scrotal tumour for five years. Their response to the newspaper article about the Calcutta Mesmeric Hospital led them to seek its assistance.[96]

On 19 September 1848, Shaikh Sulaim (Selim), a thirty-year-old husbandman, a native of Boidpatee (Baidabati), Hooghly district had been subjected to epilepsy for six years. He was cured on 2 November.[97]

Shifting to 17 November 1847, Shaikh Fyzoolla, a twenty-eight-year-old Klasse (Khalasi), a native of Hallishur (Hali Shahar) in the Chittagong district, had encountered acute rheumatism persisting for two months. Engaging in mesmerism for an hour and a half each day, he displayed notable improvement. On 11 December, he showcased the ability to walk, run, and jump similar to any other individual.[98]

Details of the Patients Treated during the Final Phase of the Calcutta Mesmeric Hospital

The final medical report of the Calcutta Mesmeric Hospital was documented in September 1948. The report outlines the details of mesmeric anaesthesia treatments conducted during that period. On 1 September, Sheik Sakroo, a forty-year-old writer, presented with a scrotal tumour of a child's head size. An operation was performed on him on 5 September 1848. Similarly, on 9 September, Mahomed Reza, a 55-year-old Khansamah, was afflicted with the same ailment.[99] Essennchunder Paul (Ishan Chandra Pal), a forty-year-old shopkeeper, arrived at the hospital on the 6th of September with a sizable tumour. His operation took place on 17 September. Approximately half an hour after the procedure, he regained full consciousness. He expressed that he had just woken up, hadn't experienced any sickness or disturbance throughout the day, had eaten and digested his breakfast as usual. The tumour's weight was measured at thirty pounds.[100] Ramsunder Dey was admitted on 3 September, presenting a scrotal tumour. Although he was prepared for surgery on the 15th, a severe fever halted the mesmeric process for two days. Eventually, the operation was performed on the 21st of September, and the tumour weighed sixteen pounds.[101]

Aged forty, Shaikh Kyratie, a *khitmutgar*, had been enduring a small tumour for twenty years. The tumour swelled significantly during fever episodes occurring once a month, causing severe pain and hindering his work. His admission was on 17 September. He underwent mesmeric trance on the first day and was operated on the 23rd of September. Towards the end of the procedure, he exhibited notable leg movements but remained asleep. As the mesmeric process continued, he returned to a state of unconsciousness. Half an hour later, he was de-mesmerised and awoke naturally, as if from sleep.[102]

Dr Esdaile provided a list of the mesmeric operations conducted at the hospitals in Hooghly and Calcutta, which is presented below:[103]

Mesmeric Anaesthetic Surgeries at the Calcutta Mesmeric Hospital

Return of Surgical Operations performed in the Calcutta Mesmeric Hospital, from November 1846 to 1st January 1848.

CASE REPORT FIRST PAGE

Diseases.	Admitted No.	Discharged.				Remarks.
		Cured.	Average period under Treatment.	Died.	Average period un-der treatment.	Remaining.
Amputation of great toe,......	1	1	76	0	0	0	This was a boy who had his toe crushed by a boat, and was in great pain, but he was deeply entranced the 1st day, and was operated on the 2d.
Amputation of Breast, ...	1	1	46	0	0	0	It weighed 7lbs.
Cartilaginous tumours of both ears removed,..	2	2	15	0	0	0	One tumour weighed 1 b., the other 5 oz. The woman was ready the first day, and was operated on the 2d.
Lithotomy,...	1	1	50	0	0	0	This man was in great pain, and was entranced the 1st day; he had hardly slept for a year.
Seirrhous testes removed,...	1	1	70	0	0	0	The parts were highly inflamed and very painful, the man was ready the 1st day, and operated on the 2d.
Sloughing testes removed,...	1	0	0	0	0	0	The man was operated on for a scrotal tumour, fever came on and caused sloughing of the testes. He was again entranced in 10 minutes, and the testes were removed, but he died a few days after.
Scrotal tumours removed,...	46	33	87	5	38	8	Of all sizes from a few lbs. to 100lbs. one on the 1st day, several on the 2d.
Total.....	53						
Case Formerly Reported.							
Abscesses opened,...	5	5	0	0	0	0	
Actual cautery applied to a sore,....	1	1	0	0	0	0	
A large sore covered with muriatic acid.....	3	3	0	0	0	0	
Carried over,...	62						

Return of Surgical Operations performed in the Calcutta Mesmeric Hospital, from November 1846 to 1st January 1848.

CASE REPORT SECOND PAGE

Diseases.	Admitted No.	Discharged.				Remaining.	Remarks.
		Cured.	Average period under Treatment.	Died.	Average period un-der treatment.		
Brought over,...	62						
Amputation of thigh,...	2	1	......	1	....	....	One was a desperate case. The right foot had sloughed off 15 days before, in consequence of having been burned with hot- red charcoal balls by a native doctor for rheumatism, and the limb was gangrenous up to the knee. He did very well for a month. The bone protruded in the other case, and he died after two months. It ought to be borne in mind that the muscles when cut across in the trance, do not contract as in the natural state, and therefore more covering than usual should be left to allow for the contraction when the patient awakes. One was operated on after two hours' mesmerising, the other within the time allowed, 24 hours.
Amputation of leg,...	1	1	...	...	....	...	Subdued the 1st day, cut off on the 4th.
Amputation of arms,...	1	1	...	...	....	....	Cut off after one hour's mesmerising.
Amputation of breast,...	1	1	...	...	....		Ditto-half an hour's do
Amputation of penis & testes,...	1	...	...	1	...	...	This was a cancer, and the man died of the constitutional disease.
Amputation of penis,...	1	...	...	1	...	...	This was also cancer, and the man died of the constitutional disease, operated on after one hour.
Amputation of testes,...	1	1	...	...	....	...	After one hour's mesmerising it was as big as a child's head, ex- quisitely painful, and complicated with rupture, which was returned in the trance.
Amputation of Scirrhous testis,	1	1	...	...	....	...	
Cancer of cheek removed,...	1	1	...	...	....	...	
Carried over,...	72						

Mesmeric Anaesthetic Surgeries at the Calcutta Mesmeric Hospital

Return of Surgical Operations performed in the Calcutta Mesmeric Hospital, from November 1846 to 1st January 1848. – (Continued)

CASE REPORT THIRD PAGE

Diseases.	Admitted No.	Discharged.		Died.	Average period un-der treatment.	Remaining.	Remarks.
		Cured.	Average period under Treatment.				
Brought over,...	72						
Cataracts operated on,...	3	3	....	....	....	....	It is a curious fact that the mesmeric trance does not facilitate operations on the eye. The eye-ball is generally turned upwards, downwards, or into either angle so far that the cornea is out of sight, or only partially visible. The eye also often rotates about the orbit so as to be with difficulty fixed. When the eye is fixed and the cornea is in front, it is often glazed like a dead man's, preventing a view of the iris. When the latter is visible, it is usually dilated or contract-ed to a pin-point, but sometimes its mobility remains. Two were operated upon on the 1st day.
End of a bone in a compound fracture sawed off,...	1	1	....	.....	.....	....	After one hour's mesmerising.
End of thumb cut off,...	1	1	....	.....	.....	....	After half an hour's mesmerising.
Fistulas laid open,..	9	9	....	.....	.....	....	Many on the first day.
Great toe nails cut out by the roots,...	5	5	....	.....	.....	....	Several ditto.
Gum cut away	1	1	....	.....	.....	....	After a few minutes' mesmerising.
Heels flayed,...	3	3	....	.....	.....	....	One on the 1st day, one on the 2d.
Hydroceles operated on,...	11	11	....	.....	.....	....	Many on the 1st day.
Hypertrophy of penis removed,...	1	1	....	.....	.....		
Hypertrophy of prepuce,	1	1	....	.....	.....	....	The first day.
Carried over,..	108						

Return of Surgical Operations performed in the Calcutta Mesmeric Hospital, from November 1846 to 1st January 1848. – (Continued)

CASE REPORT FOURTH PAGE

Diseases.	Admitted No.	Discharged.			Average period under treatment.	Remaining.	Remarks.
		Cured.	Average period under Treatment.	Died.			
Brought over,...	108						
Prolapsus ani reduced,	1	1	....	.....	.....	.....	It occurred in a man of 30, had been down for 3 days, and was as big as a child's head,–no means could reduce it. After three hours mesmerising, it was easily returned without the man knowing it.
Scrotal tumours removed,.........	25	25	.....	.....	.....	.....	Of all sizes from a few lbs. to 103 lbs., several on the 1st day.
Seton 12 inches long introduced,	1	1	....	....	.....	.....	
Straightened contracted knees	3	3	....	.....	.....	.....	
Straightened arms,	3	3	....	....	.....	.....	
Suppurating pile cut off,..	1	1	....	....	.....	.....	
Tapping for dropsy,	3	3	....	....	.....	.....	On the 1st day
Teeth extracted	5	5	....	....	.....	.....	Several on do
Tumour in the groin removed,...	1	1	....	....	.....	.....	It was found to be an undescended testis, forming a tumour the size of a moderate cauliflower. It was ulcerated and filled with maggots. The operation was performed after one hour's mesmerising.
Tumour in antrum maxillaræ ditto,...	1	1	....	....	.....	.....	It had passed under the cheek bone and orbit as far as my fingers could reach, and having destroyed the bones of the nose descended into the throat.
Tumor on leg ditto,	1	1	....	....	.....	.....	
Unhealthy sores pared down	9	9	....	....	.....	.....	Several on 1st day.
Total,...	162	152		9			

(Signed) J. ESDAILE, M.D.,
Superintendent Mesmeric Hospital.
Calcutta, Mesmeric Hospital, the 31st December, 1847.

Return of Surgical Operations performed in the Calcutta Mesmeric Hospital, from November 1846 to 1st January 1848.

CASE REPORT FIFTH PAGE

Diseases.	Number.	Discharged.				Remarks.
		Cured.	Average period under Treatment.	Relieved.	Average period Under treatment.	
Cervical glands enlarged ...	1	....	...	1	37	This girl was dreadfully disfigured, the enlarged glands preventing motion to that side altogether. All medical treatment had been useless. The swelling was reduced two-thirds in 5 weeks, when she foolishly gave up coming to the Hospital. The cure was at least happily commenced by mesmerism.
Cervical glands enlarged and painful with dimness of sight ...	1	1	2	....	....	This girl had for a great many years been subject to inflammation of the glands behind both ears, regularly twice a year, and was never relieved without suppuration of first one ear, and then the other. Leeches had been as regularly applied, and her sight had become very indistinct in consequence. The pain and enlargement disappeared in 2 days, and a few more days mesmerising quite restored her sight.
Epilepsy for 19 years...	1	1	90	...	....	Time must determine whether this lady is cured of her fits. But they have been suspended for nearly a year, and her condition much improved by being enabled to leave o leave off narcotics.
Epilepsy and insanity for 2 years,...	1	...	...	1	16	I received this man from the Lunatic Asylum. After each fit he had always become insane and violent for 8 or 10 days. He had several fits in my Hospital, but never was insane, or ill after them. He made his escape after 16 days, unluckily.
Epilepsy for 6 years,	1	....	...	1	36	This man's fits were suspended, and he insisted on going home.
Epilepsy for 9 years,	1	....	...	1	180	The fits have gradually become more irregular and less severe. After each attack the left arm was always exquisitely painful, and paralysed for several days. This has not happened lately, and he escaped monthly attack altogether last time, his case is very promising.
Carried over,...	6					

Return of Surgical Operations performed in the Calcutta Mesmeric Hospital, from November 1846 to 1st January 1848. – (Continued)

CASE REPORT SIXTH PAGE

Diseases.	Number.	Discharged.		Relieved.	Average period un-der treatment.	Remarks.
		Cured.	Average period under Treatment.			
Brought over,	6					
Epilepsy for 2 years,	1	1	49	.....	.....	This came from Lunatic Asylum.
Insensibility of the whole skin with lameness for 4 months	1	1	18	.....	.....	This man was insensible to pricking with a knife from head to foot, and walked with much difficulty.
Lameness for 5 years	1	1	5	.....	.....	
Lameness for 2 months,	1	1	24	.....	.....	
Neuralgia of half the back for a year,…	1	1	21	.....	.....	This man had been frequently scarified, leeched and blistered to no purpose.
Neuralgia from the neck to the waist for 3 months,	1	1	34	.....	.....	
Neuralgia of the spine for 4 months,	1	1	8	.....	.....	
Neuralgia and loss of power in right arm and leg for 2 months,	1	1	30	.....	.....	
Neuralgia of the stomach for 7 years,	1	....	....	1	12	This man was much relieved that he would not remain any longer.
Pain, swelling, and stiffness of the elbow for 6 mths,	1	1	10			The pain and swelling were removed, but at the ends of the bones were enlarged and prevented free motion of the joint.
Pain, weakness and partial loss of feeling in both legs, extending up to the middle for a year,	1	1	60	.....	.....	
Palsy hemiplegia,	1	....	...	1	37	Half of this man's body was powerless. When he left he was able to walk about the compound with a stick.
Palsy of left arm complete,	1	1	12	.....	.....	
Palsy partial of the right side with great weakness of the limbs for six years,......	1	1	21	.....	.....	
Carried over,...	20					

Return of Surgical Operations performed in the Calcutta Mesmeric Hospital, from November 1846 to 1st January 1848. – (Continued)
CASE REPORT SEVENTH PAGE

Diseases.	Number.	Discharged.				Remarks.
		Cured.	Average period under Treatment.	Relieved.	Average period un-der treatment	
Brought over,	20					
Palsy partial, after apoplexy, with loss of sensibility in different parts, and general muscular disability,…	1	1	60	…		
Palsy partial, paraplegia, with - loss of sensation below the loins for a month,...	1	1	10			
Rheumatism Chronic with contracted elbow joints for 5 weeks,.......	1	1	12			
Rheumatism Chronic with stiff ankle for 5 years,	1	1	30			
Rheumatism Chronic with very painful and enlarged joints and burse for two years,............	1	1	90			
Rheumatism Chronic with Acute of1 the neck, ...	1	1	1	….	…..	This man was cured by one trance.
Rheumatism Chronic Acute for 3 months,….	1	1	7	….	….	This man could not turn in bed without help.
Sciatica with lameness for 2 months,	1	1	12			
Stiff arm for 6 months, ...	1	1	43			
Stiff arm for 4 months,…	1	1	37			
Tetanus for 10 days,	1	1	30	….	….	The most active medical treatment had been of no use.
Cases formerly Reported.	1	1	..			
Convulsions,	1	1	1	….	….	The trance was induced with catalepsy in one hour.
Carried over,	32					

Return of Surgical Operations performed in the Calcutta Mesmeric Hospital, from November 1846 to 1st January 1848. – (Continued)

CASE REPORT EIGHTH PAGE

Diseases.	Number	Discharged.		Relieved.	Average period un-der treatment.	Remarks.
		Cured.	Average period under Treatment.			
Brought over,...	32					
Feeling of insects crawling body,....	1	1	1			
Nervous headaches,	3	3	1	....	....	These patients were all entranced in a very short time.
Nervousness and lameness from rheumatism for 2 years,...	1	1	30	....	....	This gentleman had made a grand tour of doctors to no purpose.
Inflammation acute of the eye,...	1	1	1	.....	.....	This man was entranced for 2 hours, sitting on a stool, twice in 24 hours; after the 2d trance, the inflammation was extinguished.
Inflammation Acute of both testes, ...	1	1	36 Hr			He was kept in the trance for 36 hours, with very short intervals of waking, and then discharged cured.
Lameness from rheumatism,...	1	1	10			
Lumbago,.........	1	1	7			
Neuralgia of crural nerve,.....	1	1	7			
Palsy of one arm,....	1	1	30			
Hemiplegia,....	1	...	...	1	42	The loss of power was complete, and he walked tolerably well when he left.
Sciatica,....	1	1	4			
Tic doloreux of long standing,...	1	1				
Total,......	46	39		7		

Calcutta, M. H. (Signed)
The 31st December, 1847. J. ESDAILE, M. D., Supt. Mes. Hospital,

(True Copy,)
J. FORSYTH, Surgeon, Secy. Medl. Board.

Over a span of eighteen months, painless mesmerism treatment continued within the confines of the Calcutta Mesmeric Hospital. Professor Allan Webb, the Demonstrative Anatomy Professor at Calcutta Medical College, assessed the approach. Information had reached him through a former student of the Medical College, confirming that Dr Esdaile had competently conducted intricate surgeries without inducing pain through the influence of mesmeric trance. This viewpoint endorsed the idea that medical practitioners should actively seek opportunities to enhance their understanding of medical science and the most effective ways to alleviate human suffering.

A new chapter unfolded in Dr Esdaile's life and the history of the Calcutta Mesmeric Hospital upon the arrival of Lord Dalhousie in India. After thoroughly reviewing accounts of painless mesmerism treatment, Lord Dalhousie was deeply impressed by Dr Esdaile's achievements.[104] As a result, an invitation was extended to Dr Esdaile to visit the Government House. Recognizing Dr Esdaile's unwavering dedication, Lord Dalhousie remarked, 'Dr Esdaile, you have no need to express gratitude to me, only to yourself. I have merely upheld justice.'[105] This pivotal development led to the appointment of Dr Esdaile as the Calcutta Presidency Surgeon. In this encouraging environment, Dr Esdaile successfully garnered support from the residents of Calcutta and other notable figures from the surrounding regions.[106]

Descent of the Enigmatic Curtain
Exploring the Final Phase of Mesmerism—Challenges and Decline

By the middle of the nineteenth century, Bengal and the rest of the world had heard about the successes of the Calcutta Mesmeric Hospital in relation to mesmeric painless surgery. According to the renowned newspaper *The Englishman*, it was opined that the recently opened Mesmeric Hospital would assist the general public by curing various maladies. Another newspaper *The Friend of India* expressed its admiration by referring to, 'The clear reluctance which the members of the committee, with one exception,' had displayed in 'acknowledging the realities proved by these experiment.' In fact *The Bombay Bi-Monthly Times* once stated that 'Dr Esdaile deserves to be ranked amongst the greatest benefactors of the human race.'[1] The governor-general had been replaced in the interim. Lord Dalhousie was appointed as the new governor-general of India. In order to verify the accuracy of the anaesthesia used during procedures, he carefully reviewed all the visitor reports made available by the hospital. There should be no doubt at all, he declared, emphasizing how pleased he was with these observations.² On 1 January 1848, Dalhousie was mentioned in *The Friend of India* as saying, 'We are pleased to note that the government has selected Dr. Esdaile as one of the Presidency Surgeons.'³ Also it stated that the government had to honour Dr Esdaile's initiative, knowledge and tenacity in furthering the use of mesmerism as a technique to lessen pain during surgery, and it did so in the most suitable manner.

An Enigmatic Paradox: The Shadow of Ambivalence in the Continuation of the Calcutta Mesmeric Hospital

Despite the success of the Mesmeric Hospital, Dalhousie did not want to continue running such a costly venture as a separate independent institution. He felt that the hospital's continuation after its tenure was quaint indulgence because it was established for one year to observe the effectiveness of mesmerism as an anaesthetic application in surgery. *The Christian Advocate*, one of the most widely read magazines at that time, stated: 'We are not prepared to say whether the government will re-establish the mesmeric hospital.' It opined that after having sanctioned the residence of Dr Esdaile with the hospital charges and appointed the doctor to a surgery in Calcutta, the Government had decided to leave, 'the native community to supply from their benevolence the current expenses of the hospital'. This meant that the hospital was to be funded by the public and not the British government. According to the *British*

Economic Correspondent, the Mesmeric Hospital's monthly expenses were allocated, and the hospital's solvency was dependent on three hundred rupees each month. At the same time, a message was sent to Calcutta's millionaires that this was a golden opportunity to prove their financial solvency.[4] They should come forward with financial help for a wonderful invention to alleviate the unbearable sufferings of the common people. At this critical juncture, instead of building bridges, wharves or excavating tanks, they invested through financial donations in nurturing the newly born Mesmeric Hospital. The appointment of Dr James Esdaile as Presidency Surgeon by Governor-General Lord Dalhousie captured the public's attention as 'an act of justice'.[5] However, it was argued, this decision was the final nail in the coffin, leaving the Mesmeric Hospital rudderless. This contradicts the assertion made by *The Englishman* which promoted a different viewpoint. It was of the opinion that the babus and so-called *bhadralok* of Calcutta, who professed their sentiment towards the Mesmeric Hospital, now had the opportunity to demonstrate their credibility by supporting the hospital financially. *Bengal Hurkaru* opined that the elite society of Calcutta would not waste any time in carrying out their responsibility, or what was believed to be their duty, in this regard. It would be pertinent to focus on the reviews of the visitors who attended painless surgical treatments through mesmeric trance. This would give one ample scope to understand the mesmeric application that in turn would help to prepare a decisive mind about the future of the Mesmeric Hospital.

Echoes of Awe: Visitors' Chronicles at the Calcutta Mesmeric Hospital

'That Brahma is above all, and Dr. Esdaile next to him,' commented Dr J.F. Mouat.[6] He taught Medical Law and Terminology at the Bengal Medical College in Calcutta. He was acknowledged as one of the Bengal Medical Service's most capable and effective employees. He had seen four of Dr Esdaile's operations first hand and discovered proof of total analgesia in each.[7] There was not even the faintest indication of physical pain throughout the surgeries. On 7 December 1847, at the beginning of the second episode, Dr Mouat wrote in complete contrast that absolute unconsciousness and insensibility to pain had been observed in only a few cases. He gave detailed information on a total of forty-nine surgical cases. Among these, complete numbness was seen in only seventeen patients, and fourteen cases were utterly numb except for minor contractures of the eyebrows and toes. Simultaneously there were thirteen cases with considerable indication of pain and five cases with failure or partial failure of the patients where they became sensitised before the operation was completed. In his report, Dr Mouat observed that mesmerism did not deserve one's confidence as a rapid, dynamic and certain agent for procuring an entirely painless operation.[8] William Brooke O'Shaughnessy also expressed his opinions concerning the use of mesmeric trance anaesthesia. He was a Royal Society of London fellow, the Assistant Surgeon of the Bengal Medical Service, and the author of *Bengal Dispensatory and Pharmacopoeia*. Beginning with 1835, he served as distinguished chemistry and natural philosophy professor at the Calcutta Medical College. He received a knighthood from Queen Victoria in 1856. He was also the inventor of modern Electric Telegraphy. He witnessed a series of painless mesmeric operations conducted by Dr Esdaile. Since the patient could not elicit the slightest physical or other indication of pain before, during, or immediately after the operation, he was fully satisfied that mesmeric trance anaesthesia could be an effective method for painless surgery.[9] Nevertheless, in his second report, Dr O'Shaughnessy gave a negative feedback on mesmeric surgical operations: 'Mesmerism can never be made available for general surgical purposes.' At the same time, ether began to be used in medicine for anaesthetic surgery. The report of Dr Ashburner about the use of ether gas had been published in *The Zoist* by Dr Elliotson. In this report he claimed that it was the most effective and quick method of anaesthetic for the human body. He said, 'It is a blessing to the human race unequalled since the first application of vaccination. It is a gas produced from Ether, inhaled through the mouth, which released a tranquil, dreamy state and an entire inaction of muscular system.'[10] O'Shaughnessy felt that with ether painless treatment would be possible without mesmerism.

Nobility's Embrace: Patronage of Mesmeric Healing by Calcutta's Elite

A group of middle-class and wealthy residents organized themselves at James Hume's house for the continuation of mesmeric surgical treatment in Calcutta. James Hume was a lawyer practising in the Calcutta Supreme Court 15 June 1839 onwards, and wrote extensively in the *Calcutta Star* newspaper. The presence of Europeans was noticeable at this gathering of the educated people of Bengali society. Raja Radhakanta Dev was the chairman of the meeting. First, Mr Hume pointed out that mesmerism was useful not only in practical medicine but also as an excellent method for physiological science. An opportunity had provided itself to study further the mesmeric truths, which Dr Esdaile now practised. The Mesmeric Hospital primarily influenced the local community of Calcutta, and they recognised it in particular and submitted a petition to the government to revive it. Babu Ramgopal Ghose read the proposed resolution and explained it to the other delegates. Dr Mouat had assumed that one mesmeriser was needed for every four patients; thus, this necessitated a hospital of 300 beds with 75 workers.[11] Keeping this in mind the elite of Calcutta put their signatures in a petition which contained a message requesting contributions of money and subscriptions to establish such a facility. It was decided that the hospital would always be open to all kinds of patients, European and native, and to all persons, regardless of caste, creed or class, who sought to cure themselves. The specifics of all medical cases would be accessible for visitors at all times, both medical and surgical. The government was also requested to afford assistance by furnishing medicines, instruments and furniture in order to establish a general dispensary along with the hospital. The delegates of this assembly such as Raja Radhakanta Dev, Rajah Suttuchurn Gosaul, Rajah Kalikishan Bahadoor, Rajah Pertub Chunder Sing, and Babu Rama Persaud Roy, H.M. Elliot, Esq., the Rev. Mr Fisher, Mr Hume, the Rev. Mr La Croix, and Dr Martin were requested to maintain co-operation with Baboo Ramgopal Ghose, the treasurer of the committee.[12]

More than 300 signatures of elite natives in Calcutta were collected to safeguard the experimental Mesmeric Hospital in Calcutta.[13] The newspapers of Calcutta were requested to publish the above resolutions and to receive donations and subscriptions for the formation and support of a mesmeric hospital in Calcutta. It was calculated that a monthly subscription of Rs 500 would be required to meet the hospital's ongoing cost. Also, it was assumed that this money could be easily raised from the members attending the meeting as all the members of the assembly belonged to the wealthy class. Some of the prominent persons were Rajah Radhakanta Dev and Rajah Kalikishan Bahadoor; Baboos Ramgopal Ghose, Rajah Pertub Chunder Sing (Pratap Chandra Sing), Rajah Nursing Chunder Roy (Narashingha Chandra Roy), Baboo Motilall Seal (Motilal Shill), Baboo Ramanoth Tagore, Baboo Promothonath Deb (Promoth Nath Dev), Baboo Debendernauth Tagore (Debendranath

Tagore), Baboo Ramgopal Ghose, Baboo Hurrymohun Sein (Hiraanmoy Sen), Madan Mohan Roy, Kumar Kalikrishna Roy, Ramprashad Roy, Ramchunder Mitter, Nundkishore Roy, Modoosooden Roy and T.H. Chatterjee; Syud Keramut Allee, and Abdool Sannud; Messrs. H.M. Elliott, Evelyn Cordon, A. Grant, J. Hume, Scott Thomson, Engledue, Wagentreiber, Martin, Blyth, Wilby, Butcher, Heatly and A. Kemp; Dr and Mr Edlin, Dr and Major Hough, Dr Webb, Fitzpatrick, and others.[14] Esdaile suggested opening the Mesmeric Hospital again from 1 July 1848, but it debuted on September 1848 and closed in September 1849. After that, Esdaile was transferred to the Sukeahs Lane Dispensary, where he continued the mesmeric practices until he left India in June 1851. He never returned to India again and died in Sydenham in 1859.[15]

Dr Esdaile resumed his mesmeric anaesthesia treatment on 1 September 1848. He confirmed to Dr Elliotson that the Mesmeric Hospital had been opened supported by public subscription. The medical instruments and furniture were provided by the government. On 6 October 1848, the *Delhi Gazette* stated, 'The mesmeric hospital is in full operation.' This hospital continued running till September 1849, and a total of sixty-eight mesmeric surgeries were performed.[16] Similar to the experimental phase, public subscription reports from September 1848 to September 1849 relating to the Calcutta Mesmeric Hospital are accessible through provincial media. During this period, the practice of mesmerism commenced when Dr Martin referred a fifty-year-old patient, Sheik Abdoolla (Sheikh Abdullah), to Dr Esdaile's Mesmeric Hospital.

The patient presented with a tumour in one eye, which had grown to cover half of his cheek. Following mesmerization on 8 October 1848, Dr Martin performed the operation in the presence of select members of the East India Company on 13 October. Notably, the patient exhibited no sensation in any part of his body during the procedure, with regular respiration and a pulse that was only marginally affected by the operation and subsequent haemorrhage. This pioneering endeavour was followed by numerous similar surgeries that leveraged mesmerism in the same year, 1848. For instance, writer Ramsoonder Doss (Ramsundar Das), aged forty-eight, had suffered from a testicular tumour for twenty years. After undergoing mesmerisation for the first time on 9 October, he successfully underwent an operation on 10 October. These cases exemplify the erstwhile application of mesmerism in surgical procedures, warranting further investigation into its historical significance and potential therapeutic applications. In this context, mesmerism refers to the induction of a hypnotic state, characterized by heightened suggestibility and a reduced sense of pain. The utilization of mesmerism in these surgical procedures suggests a burgeoning interest in the potential of hypnotic anaesthesia in the mid-nineteenth century.[17]

In a remarkable demonstration of mesmerism's anaesthetic potential, a forty-year-old cook, Bolonath, underwent surgical intervention for an enormously enlarged scrotal tumour and moderate-sized colis. His prolonged history of opium dependence, spanning eight years and eight grains of bazaar opium daily, posed no obstacle to the successful induction of mesmerisation on 10 October, which yielded natural sleep. Subsequent mesmerization sessions on 12 and 14 October rendered him insensible to fire and steel, and enabled the surgical procedure to be performed without distress, despite transient upper body movements during the operation. The patient remained oblivious to the procedure until awakening during the post-operative examination of his eyes, reporting no unusual sensations or discomfort, thereby underscoring mesmerism's profound hypnotic effects.[18] Sheikh Etawari, aged forty-two, a healthy cloth merchant, underwent mesmerism for the first time on the 18th and was operated on the 23rd. An eight-pound tumour was operated under anaesthesia with mesmeric trance, preserving all organs. He thanked Allah and then said to Esdaile very earnestly and eloquently, 'God is above all, and Esdaile is the representative of Allah on earth. Allah first gave him life, but Esdaile gave him second life and he prayed to Allah to give the golden hat to Dr. Esdaile.' Soroop Moll (Swarup Mal), aged forty, was mesmerised on the 22nd and operated on the 25th. He had a cadaveric sensation during the operation, waking up about twenty minutes after the operation. A tumour weighing eight pounds was operated on, with all organs preserved. The case of Gunga was another important one. A Hindu youth aged eighteen, Gunga came to the hospital with a broken right wrist, and swollen and weak hands. In the native hospital, mesmerism was ordered for one hour every day for the last six weeks. After three or four days, the hand swelling began to subside, the wrist became less tender each day, and at the end of six weeks, he was discharged from the hospital. On 1 February, an old woman brought her son to Dr Esdaile's hospital as a mute. The man told himself by pantomime that he possessed all powers but not the power of speech. He could not utter any words. After the first mesmerism on 2 February, he was asked if he could speak. He could then utter a single word but with great difficulty. However on 8 February he spoke with fluency and precision, and his voice was slightly weak and hoarse.[19] On 1 January 1849, *The Calcutta Star* reported a successful anaesthetised operation at the Mesmeric Hospital on the last day of December 1848. The patient was a young woman of twenty-three who had a breast tumour, and the tumour weighed ten pounds. The tumour, larger than a man's head, was attached to the body by a foot-long isthmus. It was evident that the mammary gland, the tumour, was removed without the slightest disturbance of the body from head to foot. At the end of an hour, when the informant left the hospital, she was still sleeping as tranquilly as a healthy child.

On 27 February, this same newspaper reported that Dr Esdaile had succeeded in painlessly removing a tumour weighing seventy pounds in the most successful manner. The patient came from Delhi with fourteen years of a large tumour, attracted by Dr Esdaile's fame and mesmerising trance. Dr

Esdaile took assistance from Dr Webb. It took just a couple of minutes, and after removing the tumour, the patient fainted due to massive blood loss. He was completely unaware that the operation had occurred until he was informed. His Honour Sir John Littler, Hon. Sir F. Currie, Brigadier Eckford, Major Colebrook, Captain Mayow, Captain Sayers and Dr.James Thomson and Alan Webb were present during the operation, all expressing their satisfaction at the complete success of the operation.[20] Srinath Sen, a thirty-year-old man, presented with a severe and progressively debilitating disease that had prematurely aged his physical condition to that of a fifty-year-old. He arrived at the hospital using a stick for support due to severely impaired mobility. His right leg was permanently bent outward, resisting any attempts at repositioning, and his joints were stiff and afflicted with intense pain. His frail and emaciated appearance reflected the toll of six years of suffering from a rheumatic disease, with the past two years marking a significant decline. Following fifteen days of mesmerism treatment, his condition began to improve noticeably. After two months, his legs returned to their normal position, his mobility was fully restored, and all his pain subsided. He left the hospital walking freely and in high spirits.

The other was Lunkoo, thirty-five years old, trembling for a year due to intense fever. He could not stand properly as his body trembled continuously. He could neither open nor close his hands completely. He could only raise his hands upto half of his head, and his speech was almost obscure.

He was continually kept in the condition of mesmerism for ten days. In this way, at the end of two months, he was able to walk with the help of a stick, move and open his hands to reach at the average level of the head. He could speak very well, and his body's trembling was reduced. This man was not expected to heal. Dr Esdaile was sure that physical science could not benefit him. However, it was proved that paralysis arising from old age or biological diseases was curable by mesmerism.

In the meantime, Dr Webb and Dr Esdaile went to Strong's insane asylum. There they met a prisoner. Mesmerism could, in some cases, treat the diseases of patients without surgery. The medical reports discussed so far corroborate this comment. The condition of this prisoner's hands had become very critical. His hands were swollen three times the original size, and the ulcerated fingers were constricted. Dr Strong sent him to Dr Esdaile's hospital for surgery. However, Dr Esdaile regenerated his arm without using a knife or scissors. An hour's daily application of mesmerism not only normalised the condition of the prisoner's hands but also relieved the contraction of the fingers and restored their function.[21] Sheikh Buckak, a forty-year-old man, had neuralgia for two months. He felt it was better to die than to endure such severe headaches. He was discharged on being cured after twenty days of mesmerising. Ali Khan, twenty-six years of age, also suffered from sciatica for eight months. His legs became stiff, and he could not lead a normal life due to severe pain. He was cured in a month through mesmeric trance. Everything was going well. In the meantime, a severe economic crisis broke out in Calcutta.

Fractured Foundations: Economic Quandaries and Withdrawal of the Elites of Calcutta

On 5 September 1849, Dr Esdaile informed Dr Elliotson through a letter that the collapse of the Union Bank was the cause of a severe economic crisis in Calcutta.[22] As a result, he wrote, most of Calcutta's people faced tremendous suffering. At the same time, Calcutta's elite and influential people were busy dealing with the disaster, and finding a solution for it. As a result, the Mesmeric Hospital was cut off from the support it had received from the elite society of Calcutta.[23] From this point onwards, the Calcutta Mesmeric Hospital was gradually distanced from the core focus of Calcutta's elites. At this point, Dr Esdaile assumed that it would no longer be reasonable to defend the hospital's future plans based on public subscription. So he thought of continuing the practice of mesmerism through the Sukeahs Lane Hospital and Dispensary under government instructions and joined as superintendent of this hospital on 25 March 1851.[24]

On 9 April 1850, the *Calcutta Morning Chronicle* wrote about government backing for the Mesmeric Hospital. Dr Esdaile informed the subscribers that he would not require an extension of their liberality beyond the current month, as the Sukeahs Lane Hospital and Dispensary had been put at his disposal for the express purpose of introducing mesmerism into regular hospital practice. The only extant account of mesmerism in Calcutta after Esdaile's departure is an article titled 'An Account of the Mesmeric Hospital in Bengal since Dr. Esdaile's Departure from India', published in *The Zoist* No. XXXIX in October 1852. This article, communicated by Dr Elliotson, reveals that the Sukeahs Lane hospital continued to operate under the leadership of Dr Webb, catering to the general public. Purmanund Set, Sub-Assistant Surgeon, submitted a report highlighting the hospital's enhanced reputation and utility, which had garnered the trust of affluent patients seeking mesmerism-induced surgical interventions. These individuals were willing to incur the full costs of their treatment and remain as in-patients, a testament to the institution's burgeoning reputation. On occasions, distinguished persons opted to undergo mesmerism-induced surgeries, shouldering the expenses of their own care. Notable examples include Gopul Chunder Bose, a scribe with the Bengal Secretariat; Rammohun Roy, a merchant; Isser Chunder Sircar, a merchant; and Nufferloll Ghosain, a priest to His Highness the Maharajah of Burdwan, all of whom demonstrated their confidence in the hospital's expertise. However, following this article, there is a dearth of recorded evidence of mesmerism's application in colonial Bengal, suggesting a decline in interest in the practice.[25]

Chloroform's Curtain Call: Mesmerism's Twilight and the Rise of Western Medicine

Doctor Simpson first used chloroform in Edinburgh on 15 November 1847, and the first chloroform anaesthesia, that is the world's first ether anaesthesia, was administered on 16 October 1846, in Boston, USA. Under the supervision of surgeon Dr O'Shaughnessy, the first administration of ether anaesthesia in India was on Monday, 22 March 1847, at the Medical College Hospital, Calcutta. The first chloroform anaesthesia was administered in India on 12 January 1848. David Waldie, a chemist from Calcutta, is credited with introducing chloroform to clinical anaesthesia in Calcutta in 1853.[26] He also started his chemical company and lived there until he died in 1889. In 1888, Edward Lawrie in Hyderabad claimed to have administered chloroform anaesthesia to 40,000 people without a single death and formed the First Hyderabad Chloroform Commission of which Patrick Hehir was the president. He published his report in April 1893.[27] One hundred and forty-one animals were tested. It was concluded that 'Chloroform can be given perfectly safely and without fear of accidental death, only if care is taken in respiration.' Unfortunately, his report had not been accepted by the Medical Board of England; hence, the Second Hyderabad Chloroform Commission was formed to investigate the same.

In the UK, surgeons Laurie and Rustamji performed side-by-side experiments on 430 animals (dogs, monkeys, horses, goats, rats, rabbits and cats) and conducted a clinical study on fifty-four humans. They concluded that the Edinburgh School was correct. This research was done at Afzalganj Hospital in Hyderabad, where the Osmania Hospital is now present. Incidentally, the first female anaesthetist in India and perhaps the world, Rupbai Ferdunji, was working under Edward Lawrie in Hyderabad in 1889. Later, she went to Edinburgh for further studies. However, during the first sixteen years of chloroform anaesthesia, 393 deaths were reported, and forty-eight were reported due to ether. A controversy affected the two medical schools, with Simpson in Edinburgh claiming death from respiratory failure and John Snow in London claiming cardiac failure as the cause of death. A similar committee set up by the British Medical Association in 1875 reported five years later that chloroform was much more injurious to the heart than ether. The British Medical Association appointed the Glasgow Committee in 1880. It was therefore a blow to the London school when the so-called Hyderabad Commissions of 1889 and 1891 reported in favour of the 'clinical' school in Edinburgh.[28] The British Medical Association refused to accept their findings and set up another committee in 1891, which reported in the vaguest of terms ten years later that, 'Chloroform is injurious to the heart and more dangerous than ether in comparison.'[29]

In 1890, with twenty years of accidents caused by chloroform, a firm decision was taken against its use. Later, around the world, chloroform began to be phased out in favour of ether. However, since the beginning of the twentieth century, chloroform has become a favourite of doctors in painless surgery. One notable instance illustrating the widespread use of chloroform in medical procedures during the early twentieth century occurred when Mahatma

Gandhi was incarcerated in Yeravda Jail. On 12 January 1924, Gandhi underwent an emergency appendectomy at Sassoon Hospital in Pune. The operation was performed by British Colonel Surgeon Maddock, a prominent figure in the medical field of the time. To ensure Gandhi remained free of pain throughout the procedure, Dr Date, the chief anaesthesiologist, administered open-drop chloroform anaesthesia. This historical event underscores the prevalent reliance on chloroform as an anaesthetic agent during that period, reflecting its significant role in surgical practices.[30] Till 1928 chloroform was the only anaesthetic used in India. 'Chloroformed' was the popular expression for anaesthesia because it was cheap and easy. Dr Jyoti Prasad of Jodhpur produced a classic documented paper in 1928 on ether and observed that open ether was practical; it was cost effective even in hot weather.

The discovery of ether and chloroform was a significant obstacle to mesmerism. Earlier, the breakthrough method of insensible surgery was mesmerism, brought to India by James Esdaile. However, with the arrival of ether and chloroform in India, several weaknesses of mesmerism became a matter of discussion in medical circles. Not every person was able to induce unconsciousness by mesmerism, nor every patient susceptible to mesmeric effects. However, in the case of chloroform the result was certain as once the patient was administered with it he/she fell into a state of unconsciousness. Hence, ether and chloroform gradually became the doctors' only means of painless surgery. Dr O'Shaughnessy, in his report on the Mesmeric Hospital, commented, 'I look upon mesmerism as no longer worthy of the serious consideration of the operating surgeon.' Dr Duncan Stewart advised, 'It is the time to throw away mummery and work above board, now we have got ether.'[31] Chloroform was much more certain but could not be said to be risk-free. Mr Bennett, in the *Edinburgh Monthly Journal*, says, 'The poisonous action of Chloroform, as observed in animals, is precisely similar to that of a pure narcotic.' The *Medical Gazette*, July 1848 reported, 'The poison enters at once into the circulation and penetrates through the whole system, but there is a few minutes elapse between apparently perfect health and the death of the patient. Art is powerless in dealing with the poisonous effects of the vapour.'

In a paper 'On Death from Chloroform', Mr Sibson says, that when asphyxia is induced, 'we must regard chloroform as one of the most uncontrollable narcotic poisons but to proceed to its effects upon man. If the following people were not poisoned, I should like to know what happened to them:—

> A lady at Boulogne, 30 years of age, in good health, was put under the influence of chloroform to have a small abscess in the thigh opened. A handkerchief with fifteen or twenty drops of chloroform was held under the nostrils. The patient only made a few inspirations, when she cried, 'I'm suffocating and died on the instant.

A dentist in London gave a healthy looking young man chloroform to inhale. After six inspirations his head dropped, and he never moved or spoke after. A lady at Cincinnati, died at the expiration of five minutes after inhaling chloroform. She was in excellent health. In the case at Hyderabad, the operating surgeon reports that 'the death was almost instantaneous'. At the hospital Beaujon in Paris, M. Robert had only made one flap in a case of amputation when the patient died. Mr. Spencer Wells reports, 'I saw a patient die in bed just as M. Malgaine had completed disarticulation at the shoulder joint, and feel convinced that chloroform was the immediate cause of death.' A druggist's boy in Aberdeen was found dead, leaning upon the counter with his face in a towel, which he had impregnated with chloroform. A girl at Newcastle died in two minutes after inhaling chloroform for the removal of a toe-nail. Having only one medical periodical at hand, I know not how many more fatal cases may have been reported elsewhere, but enough has been said for my purpose, and it is to be hoped that we shall hear no more of the innocuous nature of chloroform. It would fill a whole number of your Journal to notice the disagreeable and dangerous after effects of chloroform.[32]

On the other hand, Dr Esdaile's success in treating unconscious persons with mesmerism, even the critical ones, increased with practice. He was also happy to report that no one had ever seen any harmful symptoms following a mesmeric trance for surgical purposes. He claimed that hundreds and thousands of visitors in the city of Calcutta could testify to this, and he mentioned ample names of doctors who had witnessed his mesmeric operations. He opined that physicians ought to hate themselves if, from mere sensibility and avarice, he continued to induce the public to spend their money to support an old system. If there were any doubts among the public and the medical profession in India as to the superiority of mesmerism over all drugs applied to induce insensibility to pain, he said, he would be glad at any time to demonstrate the relative truth. Even if some completely side-effect-free drug eliminated mesmerism for surgical purposes, the operation would still greatly serve surgeons in treating surgical diseases. For by this, he would often be able to save his patients from much pain and distress while curing them. Often they were spared a painful treatment to save their lives. While many had little or no pain after the operation, others suffered severely after an interval. However, being in mesmerism, it was possible to extinguish the pain in a few minutes, to which two committee members, Dr Martin and Rev. Mr La Croix, testified. According to Dr Esdaile, if any persons in Calcutta still disbelieved in the reality of painlessness under mesmeric operations, it was due to ignorance of knowledge and fear of correcting their accurate judgments by the evidence of their senses. They had been publicly invited to come and invigilate the mesmeric experiment.[33]

Metamorphosis Unveiled: Western Ascendancy and Calcutta's New Medical Landscape

Mesmerism, on the one hand, was easily accessible for the common person. On the other hand, though mesmerism did not require any medicinal treatment, it emerged as a new competitor in the Western drug market. The end of the nineteenth century marks the beginning of the time when there have been the largest number of changes to both the character of state government policies and the medical profession. This transition was brought about by the emergence of an English-speaking class of Indians who served as the backbone of the nationalist movement, as well as by increasingly prosperous traders, significant landowners, and new industries. Both indigenous and Western medical practitioners evolved towards a professional paradigm over the years 1860–1920.[34] The demand of a Western-educated middle class who preferred Western medicines led to the establishment of the Calcutta-based Western drugs market. Western medicine and the drug market emerged around the Calcutta Medical College in the mid-nineteenth century. Professionalization of medicine in India represented colonial attempts to carry over the medical practices of an industrial society into a vastly different developing society. The Western medicine market gradually developed as 'Colonial Enclaves'.[35] Early East India Company sergeants mainly depended on indigenous Indian medicine for treatment, commonly known as 'bazar medicine'. It was in the interest of the imperialists that the city was hygienic and that diseases and epidemics were controlled. Hence, they used both imposition and accommodation to bring the citizens within the Western purview of medicine and hygiene. They tried to impress upon the natives that the body is not a mere appendage to the soul. They harped on how it was a functional system where ailments could be treated by systematic investigations, medicines and surgeries. Thus, they introduced the natives to Western modernity. This success was always assessed by the colonisers as one of their greatest achievements.[36] An assortment of Western medicines was accessible through local vendors specializing in indigenous remedies, many of whom also traded in spices. In Bengal, these indigenous or bazaar medicines, as they were interchangeably termed, became a consistent source for English military hospitals by the mid-eighteenth century. Simultaneously they sold medicinal plants and herbs with other commercial products to connect with the rural people and fulfilled their medicinal requirements. So the end of mesmeric surgery unquestionably freed the Western drug market from a great deal of competition on the one hand while, on the other hand, by labelling the mesmeric process as superstitious, it was the perfect opportunity for the British to charge up their Western civilising mission for this action. The British government had always endeavoured to uphold Western scientific thought at the highest level. Therefore they were unwilling to accept mesmerism as a method of treatment, which was thought of as a 'Mystical Witch from the birth time'.

However, Dr Esdaile defended mesmerism for the treatment of various ailments with his own argument. He concluded that 'if the proud sons of the civilisation will condescend to return for a moment to the feet of their mother nature, they also will probably benefit by her bounties'.[37] Dr Esdaile was always enthusiastic about demonstrating his invention to Calcutta's middle and upper classes. But the British government speculated that mesmeric trance was a magical process or more of a chimera, which must have been the reason for the increased popularity of Dr Esdaile's mesmerism treatment in Bengal.[38] In this context, this idea became vital that mesmerism was more superstition than science, and perceived as a supernatural power by the public. According to the British government, those who went to Dr Esdaile's hospital were attracted only by his fame, which was obtained through mesmeric trance, and they flocked to him impressed with the fullest and firmest beliefs in his supernatural powers. The common people believed in the existence and activity of an 'invisible remedy'.[39] The British authorities attempted to create a link between the mesmeric anaesthetic application with occultism, and its first practitioner in India, Dr James Esdaile, with a magician. They said that when Dr Esdaile first came to Bengal, he had the honour of being introduced to one of the most famous magicians in Bengal, known widely for his successful treatment of hysteria. In fact, Esdaile had once introduced himself as a magician's brother who had studied the art of magic in different parts of the world.[40]

Mystique and Modernity: Revelation of the Preconceived Notions of the Bengali Mindset and the Sanctity of Mesmerism

This section delineates the growing resonance of Dr James Esdaile's reputation within the British colonial landscape, particularly in the context of Bengal. This phenomenon can be attributed to the prevailing belief among the Bengali population in Esdaile's purported supernatural healing prowess. The Bengalis demonstrated a remarkable capacity for harmonizing their pre-existing cognitive frameworks with Esdaile's prescribed therapeutic regimen, which included confinement within a dimly lit chamber. Consequently, the Mesmeric Hospital led by Esdaile underwent a semantic shift, colloquially acquiring the moniker Jadoo Hospital or the House of Magic.[41] This nomenclature serves to underscore the perception of a mystical and enigmatic quality inherent in the curative procedures conducted within its walls. This transformation, from a conventional medical facility to a perceived locus of magical intervention, offers a nuanced lens through which one can comprehend the intricate interplay of cultural beliefs, colonial dynamics, and evolving medical paradigms during this historical epoch.

The British government was surprised by the acceptance of mesmeric anaesthesia among the Bengalis. It tried to break down a superstitious, closed society in mid-nineteenth-century Calcutta and create a new mould wrapped in the mantle of Western modernity.[42] The idea of painless surgery, by connecting the magician with the idea of supernatural power, became a cause of fear for the Western powers.

Thus, it is seen that the Mesmeric Hospital in Calcutta instituted by Dr James Esdaile was not exempt from the lustful gaze of Western imperialism. Despite being a groundbreaking development at the time, the British government was not reluctant to correlate mysticism with the mesmeric process because it went against their commercial interests. As a consequence, the East India Company dismantled the Mesmeric Hospital and replaced it with the Western drug that was marketed while valuable chloroform was used to promote Western excellence. However, in addition to the colonial invasion, the advent of chloroform and its use in medicine, the economic depression affected the elite of Calcutta, thereby producing an unfavourable climate for mesmerism in the city, which ultimately resulted in the demise of the Calcutta Mesmeric Hospital.

Nevertheless, viewing the above-mentioned reasons as the sole and primary cause for the cessation of mesmerism and the closure of the Calcutta Mesmeric Hospital should not be accepted without scrutiny. It is irrefutable that Western capitalism exerted a considerable influence over the domain of mesmerism. However, this was not the sole impediment encountered by the contemporaneous medical community when confronted with the concept of a non-pharmacological, painless surgical procedure. One of the foremost challenges mesmerism faced was its perceived lack of universality. Several European surgeons contended that the application of mesmerism's techniques did not yield consistent results across all populations. According to them, mesmerism's efficacy appeared to be largely confined to the native inhabitants of Bengal, with comparatively limited impact on Europeans and Eurasians. Dr Thomson, in particular, articulated a principled objection to the utilization of mesmerism in surgical contexts, positing that while it exhibited notable success among the natives, its effectiveness remained uncertain and often resulted in complete failure when administered to individuals of European and Eurasian descent. This uncertainty extended to the duration required to induce a deep mesmeric sleep. It is worth noting that the surge in popularity and acclaim enjoyed by Esdaile in Bengal contributed to a widespread belief in his extraordinary or supernatural abilities among the general populace, thus further complicating the discourse surrounding mesmerism.[43] Interestingly, Dr Thomson, in spite of his critique, preferred the application of mesmeric trance over that of sulphuric ether.

An additional contributing factor to the multifaceted discourse surrounding mesmerism resides in its association with the supernatural. Notably, Esdaile himself forged a conceptual linkage between mesmerism and the domain of magic, thereby establishing a correlation between the requisite darkened environment and the necessary altered physical state for the practice of mesmerism. This inherent connection effectively interwove mesmerism with the rich tapestry of magical traditions that permeated the cultural milieu of the Bengal region. From the vantage point of European surgeons, the prevailing popularity of the Calcutta Mesmeric Hospital predominantly hinged upon the prevalence of superstitious beliefs among the indigenous populace of Bengal. A profound and unswerving faith in the efficacy of magic, coupled with the perceived miraculous prowess of the attending physician, formed the bedrock of the collective belief in the healing potential inherent in mesmerism. Dr Mouat, for example, made observations underscoring mesmerism's capacity to ameliorate a spectrum of functional disorders within the realms of the nervous and vascular systems. He opined that few populations across the globe exhibited such profound susceptibility to superstition, manifesting in a comprehensive and occasionally seemingly irrational manner, as was discernible within the native demographic of Bengal. This prevailing undercurrent of belief in witchcraft and the omnipotence of occult practices permeated the collective psyche with unwavering conviction. It is evident from numerous entries within the annals of medical records that this reservoir of faith and belief significantly influenced the mitigation of both spiritual and physiological afflictions within the domains of the nervous and vascular systems.[44]

The effectiveness of mesmerisers in the practice of mesmerism was far from uniform, with significant variation observed among practitioners despite their training. During this period, trained native doctors, while possessing some training, often lacked the proficiency required for the accurate application of mesmerism. It is notable that only a limited cadre of physicians exhibited genuine interest in embracing this therapeutic modality. It is worth emphasizing that, within the context of a medical facility housing 300 beds, a staggering seventy-five mesmerisers would be necessary to adequately allocate one mesmeriser for every four patients.[45] This disparity underscores the formidable demand for skilled practitioners in the field of mesmerism. However, it is essential to contextualize this challenge within the evolving societal landscape of Bengal during this era. A discernible shift was occurring wherein individuals holding certifications in Western medical science were increasingly gaining prominence within the aristocratic strata of Bengali society. Consequently, there was a gradual transformation in the perception of Western-trained doctors as being of greater importance. This transition contributed to the emergence of a marked shortage of mesmerisers, thus casting an aura of uncertainty over the sustained practice of mesmerism within the medical domain. The interplay of these factors, including the varied effectiveness of mesmerisers, the limited interest of physicians in this method, and the evolving medical landscape of Bengal, collectively engendered an intricate situation for the continued utilization of mesmerism as a therapeutic modality.

The endorsement of mesmerism was met with notable objection, particularly within the framework of medical ethics. There existed considerable uncertainty regarding the extent to which mesmerism could induce a profound state of unconsciousness in the patient. Reports from attending physicians frequently indicated that certain sensations and susceptibilities to pain endured during surgical procedures, even under the influence of mesmerism. Medical practice steadfastly upholds the principle of never reawakening a patient once rendered unconscious, while surgical intervention necessitates the contrary course of action. It was not infrequent for patients to regain consciousness midway through the operation, thereby exacerbating their distress and agony.

Moreover, the application of mesmerism was encumbered by significant temporal constraints. The duration required to elicit insensibility was protracted; certain cases mandated extensive trials spanning several days, ranging from one to as many as six to eight, to achieve the desired attenuation of sensory perception. This rendered mesmerism ill-suited for exigencies where the imperative for immediate intervention precluded the luxury of time. Dr Richard O'Shaughnessy, a practitioner affiliated with the Medical College, vociferously opposed the integration of mesmerism into surgical practice, deeming it an antiquated method antedating the advent of ether. Dr O'Shaughnessy contended that, in light of the availability of ether—a pharmacological agent with well-understood potency, virtually assured efficacy, and a track record of proven harmlessness in the alleviation of surgical pain—mesmerism was to be regarded with heightened gravity. Its judicious application rested solely within the purview of the operating surgeon, contingent upon the patient's stable physiological state devoid of pain or constitutional disruptions, such as fever. Bleeding during mesmerised surgery mirrored the profuseness observed in conventional procedures, prompting apprehensions regarding the prospect of untimely arousal. Additionally, the requisite preoperative examination imposed an injurious toll on the operator's well-being, compelling expedited procedures. Dr O'Shaughnessy adjudged ether to be the more dependable option, as it demonstrated equal if not superior efficacy, adaptable to diverse auditory environments, whether clamorous or subdued.[46] In juxtaposition to mesmerism's inherent limitations, ether emerged as a preeminent choice for surgical anaesthesia, underscoring its unequivocal efficacy and expedience.

In the early stages of anaesthesia, chloroform encountered several adverse outcomes, as documented in Sibson's account of unsuccessful treatment with this agent, which has already been mentioned. In response to Sibson's remarks, O'Shaughnessy asserted:

> The dangers are imaginary. The reported fatal effects attributed to ether, all practical men now laugh at. Yet everybody knows that within a year from its discovery, fatal ether cases had become so numerous that it became absolutely necessary to seek some safer general anaesthetic agent, and hence the birth of chloroform, destined apparently to an equally short universal empire. If the Professor of Surgery expects us to respect him as an authority, his opinions will be better considered and

his statements more correct in future when writing in a Medical Journal, or reporting to Government upon a scientific subject. Such Delphic responses may overawe and impose upon an audience of Hindoo boys, but are only calculated to make 'all practical men laugh.'... Ether and chloroform for surgical purposes are most valuable additions to our armoury, and, I believe, that I was the first individual in this country who tested their powers.

While the efficacy of mesmerism faced a barrage of inquiries in subsequent assessments, it is undeniable that it stood as a remarkable and extraordinary revelation of the antiquated ethereal epoch. To the medical milieu of yore, the notion of assuaging physical anguish amidst surgical interventions appeared nigh implausible. Yet, within the domain of mesmerism, lay the potentiality for conducting surgical procedures devoid of pharmacological interventions, thereby heralding the prospect of painless surgical experiences. However, its incongruity with the contemporaneous epoch posed a formidable challenge to its veracity, ultimately culminating in its obsolescence within colonial Bengal. The evolving exigencies and advancements of the era precipitated a re-evaluation of mesmerism's applicability, rendering it progressively incongruent with the evolving paradigms of medical practice. This shift in perspective and the escalating reliance on more contemporary therapeutic modalities ultimately led to the eclipse of mesmerism's once prominent status within the medical landscape of colonial Bengal.

Mesmerism's Legacies
Power Dynamics, Cultural Exchange, and the Blurring of Scientific and Non-Scientific Practices with Special Focus on the Theosophical Society

The nineteenth century was a period of fusion of Eastern and Western medical models that created the background of mesmerism in Calcutta. Dr James Esdaile's effort in mesmerism's application through the Calcutta Mesmeric Hospital is most significant. In colonial Calcutta, mesmerism was the first method used for pain manipulation during surgery, and it progressively gained popularity among the Bengalis.

However a shadow of ambivalence in the continuation of the Calcutta Mesmeric Hospital came with the spread of Western medicine in colonial Calcutta, specially with chloroform as an agent for anaesthetic surgery. The dawn of the colonial empire and the West's extravagant trends triumphed over the East. The Bengalis underwent not only political and economic transitions but also intellectual, ideological and identity exchanges. As a result, the ideas and tastes of the Bengalis also changed to reflect the West's 'modern civilized' legacy. The East India Company then speculated about transforming Calcutta into a European town. New philosophies were launched in order to achieve their goal. At the commencement of this civilizing movement, the existence of the inhabitants was demolished. Western philosophies, education, attire, and manners introduced a 'civilized' revolution to Calcutta. The list of civilized components also included Western medical research. Western imperialism hastily sought out new drug markets for the Western pharmaceutical industry under the guise of modernity.

The Calcutta Mesmeric Hospital was ordered to close down on the pretext of linking it with superstition and supernatural powers. Even after the positive reviews of the professors of the Calcutta Medical College who pointed out the effectiveness of the mesmeric process, the efficacy of mesmerism was questioned. The main reason was the attempt to capture the Western medicine market. However, the hospital was run for a period of time with private subscriptions from the wealthy elites of Calcutta at the time. But economic distress and the discovery of chloroform ensured the virtual end of mesmerism. Eventually, mesmerism was denounced in derogatory terms associating it with magic and supernatural powers, which was said to be the main reason for its popularity among the people of Calcutta. Thus, the use of mesmeric anaesthesia during surgery gradually faded away from the early medical history of colonial Calcutta.

Though mesmerism died out in the turmoil caused by the invasion of Western imperialism, several factors prevented this astounding medical practice from being lost forever. In this instance, Bengal was already affected by a cholera outbreak, and death processions could be witnessed everywhere. The patients desperately sought medical attention but there was a scarcity of doctors certified in Western medicine to meet this demand. It was observed that the Vernacular Licentiate in Medical Service (VLMS) then began to fill this gap which led to the resumption of Western medical practice in the local language.[1] The Calcutta Medical School, which was exclusively operated by Indians, was founded in 1886 alongside the Western medical institution. Meanwhile Hakim Ajmal Khan revitalised Ayurvedic medicine in India during the last decade of the nineteenth century.

Government policy towards the medical profession and the state was transformed, with its origins in the late nineteenth century. In the Indian medical system, both native-born and foreign-born physicians developed a professional model of medical culture between 1860 and 1920. An English-speaking class that arose in Calcutta served as the backbone of the nationalist movement and laid the foundation for the emergence of new industrialists, prosperous business persons, and wealthy landowners. In the latter decades of the nineteenth century, charitable dispensaries were established in Bengal. Local panchayats and municipalities were mandated to bring *vaidya*s and *hakim*s into the fold of Western medical treatment. In the nineteenth century, the notion and structure of medical care appeared to have evolved. Hospital medicine, which was now the most popular model for public health, concentrated on the symptoms and signs that together made up a pathology.

Theosophical Society and Mesmerism: Observational Medicine, Power Struggles, and Nationalist Surge in Colonial Calcutta

In the mid-nineteenth century, following the demise of Dr Esdaile's mesmerist practices, the discipline underwent a dichotomous development, bifurcating into two distinct branches: spiritualism and hypnotism. Spiritualism, which acknowledged the extrasensory capabilities of the fluidic medium, flourished initially in North America before migrating to England in a modified form. Conversely, hypnotism evolved into a therapeutically oriented medical procedure, focusing on the treatment of physico-psychological disorders with scientifically explicable origins.

The theosophists' contributions to the popularization of mesmerism and hypnotism in post-Esdaile India were significant. Notably, the Theosophical Society, founded in New York in November 1875 by Helena Petrovna von Hahn Blavatsky (1831-1891), Colonel Henry Steel Olcott (1831-1907), and others, played a pivotal role in perpetuating the spiritual connotations of mesmerism. Madame Blavatsky and Colonel Olcott's teachings on the curative powers of mesmerism and hypnotism resonated with Indian intellectuals and spiritual seekers. As the society's influence grew in India, especially after its relocation to Adyar in 1882, theosophists like Annie Besant and Col. Steel Olcott actively promoted the practice of mesmerism and hypnotism as a means to harness human natural energies for spiritual growth, healing, and self-improvement. This led to a surge in the interest in mesmerism and hypnotism among Indian enthusiasts, who saw these practices as a way to reconcile traditional Indian spiritual beliefs with modern scientific discoveries. By the early twentieth century, mesmerism and hypnotism had become integral parts of India's spiritual and cultural landscape, with many Indian practitioners incorporating these techniques into their spiritual and therapeutic practices.[2]

The Tagores of Jorasanko were notably open-minded towards mesmerism, with many of them showing a serious interest in theosophy.[3] Prominent figures like Madame Blavatsky and Col. Henry Steel Olcott often visited the Jorasanko residence. In April 1882, the Ladies' Theosophical Society was established in Calcutta, with Mrs Alice Gordon as president and Mrs Swarnakumari Devi Ghosal, the daughter of Devendranath Tagore, as secretary. This initiative led to the founding of the newspaper *Bharati*.[4] Swarnakumari Devi (1855-1932), the tenth child of Devendranath Tagore and the sister of Rabindranath Tagore, became a leading proponent of mesmerism in Bengal during this period. Swarnakumari was a well-known writer who played a key role in bringing attention to issues affecting women and children in the early years of the nationalist movement. Her historical novel *Hooghlyr Imambari* (1884) was an important work for understanding the Hooghly Imambarah, the birthplace of mesmerism in India. Married at the age of twelve to Janakinath Ghosal, a Positivist and member of the Theosophical Society, Swarnakumari was encouraged by her husband to discard the *purdah*, which allowed her to pursue writing and social work. She became a prominent writer and editor, managing the literary monthly *Bharati* for thirty years. Her interest in mesmerism is evident in her writings from 1885 to 1894. In 1885, Swarnakumari wrote a three-part series titled '*Indriyer Sahajya Bina Moner Kotha Jana*' (Mind-Reading Without Sensory Assistance), which demonstrates her stance towards mind-reading as scientifically questionable, despite her goal of proving its scientific validity. Her belief in mind-reading and mesmerism was influenced by her predecessors. She aimed to support the idea of a suprasensory phenomenon with scientific evidence. Her work discusses the latest developments in Western psychical research from a believer's perspective, critiquing Dr James Braid's hypnotism theories and arguing for an extrasomatic force similar to Mesmer's animal magnetism. Swarnakumari Devi draws on her personal experience with a teenage boy who demonstrated trance-inducing abilities, showcasing her intellectual engagement with the debates surrounding mesmerism and hypnotism.

The following year, in 1886, she wrote a four-part series on mesmerism, reflecting the growing curiosity about this topic in Bengal. Throughout the series, she aimed to validate mesmerism over James Braid's concept of hypnotism, despite Braid's scientific explanation of trance. She believed that only a mesmeric explanation, which included the idea of an invisible fluidic medium, could account for extraordinary phenomena such as extrasensory communication, based on the evidence gathered by a nascent society for research into the 'paranormal', namely the Society for Psychical Research. As the editor of *Bharati*, Swarnakumari also edited two articles on animal magnetism or *jantob chumbakshakti*.[5] Swarnakumari Devi's oeuvre serves as a paradigmatic exemplar of the profound impact of mesmerism's spiritual and suprasensory dimensions on Indian thought during the late nineteenth century. Her literary and editorial endeavours, particularly in the literary monthly *Bharati*, substantially contributed to the discourse on mesmerism, spiritualism, and theosophy, thereby shaping the intellectual topography of Bengal and beyond. Concurrently, two other members of the Philosophical Society, Col. H.S. Olcott and Annie Besant, were profoundly influenced by mesmerism, with the former achieving renown as a distinguished mesmerist.

Mesmerism in Bengali Literature: A Critical Exploration of how Bengali Writers Shaped the Public Understanding of Mesmerism

Beyond the confines of institutional frameworks, mesmerism also permeated the literary landscape of nineteenth and twentieth-century Bengal, with notable writers incorporating its concepts and ideas into their works. Bankim Chandra Chattopadhyay's novels *Chandrashekhar* and *Rajani* serve as exemplary instances. In *Chandrasekhar*, the author dedicates the seventh section to Yogi Ramananda Sanyasi's explication of Shaivalini's psychotherapy and psychic force, demonstrating a clear engagement with mesmerist principles. Furthermore, in the sixth chapter of the sixth volume, Chattopadhyay alludes to spiritually empowered water, reminiscent of the magnetized water central to mesmerist practices. This literary integration of mesmerism underscores its pervasive influence on Bengali intellectual and cultural circles during this period. In *Rajani*, the character Sachindra is thoroughly mesmerised by the sanyasi, resulting in a hypnotic state where he perceives a blind flower girl. In the fourth volume's fifth section, Sachindra provides a detailed account of his mesmeric trance, describing his inability to articulate what he sees despite being able to perceive external objects with his eyes open. Through Sachindra's narrative, Bankim Chandra critiques the limitations of conventional medicine in addressing psychological ailments, implying the superiority of mesmerist techniques in this realm.

In his literary work *Madhavi Kankan* Rameshchandra Dutt, a prominent economic historian of India, explores the concept of mesmerism through a compelling narrative featuring the character Narendra. This anecdote exemplifies the author's interest in mesmerist techniques and their potential applications in psychotherapy. By weaving mesmerism into his literary narrative, Dutt participates in the ongoing dialogue about mental health and psychotherapy during that period, underscoring the significant cultural and intellectual impact of mesmerism on Indian thought. Prabhat Kumar Mukhopadhyay (1873-1932), a distinguished short story writer of the nineteenth century, exhibits a notable engagement with mesmerism in his literary oeuvre. His fourth volume of collected short stories explicitly addresses mesmerism, while his novels *Chandrasekhar* and *Jogobal na Psychic Force?* delve deeper into the subject. The latter work features Sabatini, a renowned mesmerist of the time, whose fame is global and unparalleled. As Mukhopadhyay writes, 'The news spread that an Italian gentleman named Sabatini, a master of hypnotism, had arrived at the Grand Hotel in Calcutta, capable of curing various ailments through hypnotism.'[6]

The novel, functioning as a literary mirror, reflects a deliberately constructed and fragmented image of society, influencing readers' perceptions and creating a mental representation that may diverge from the author's intentions. This disparity between the author's vision and the reader's interpretation precipitates a new chapter of critical engagement, as readers strive to reconcile the presented image with their own understanding of the world, thereby fostering a deeper exploration of the text and its meanings. Prabhat Kumar Mukhopadhyay's portrayal of mesmerism in his novel perpetuates a misguided understanding of the phenomenon, likely to mislead readers. The character of Navagopala, a wealthy Calcutta elite, exemplifies this misconception. Despite expressing interest in mesmerism, Navagopala relies on Bankim Chandra's fictional works *Chandrasekhar* and *Rajani* rather than scholarly texts by James Esdaile, John Elliotson and James Braid. This conflation of mesmerism with hypnosis, as depicted in Bankim Chandra's novels, led to a misguided understanding among early supporters of mesmerism in Calcutta, exemplified by Navagopala's character. Mukhopadhyay's portrayal highlights the detrimental impact of literary representations on public understanding, perpetuating misconceptions and obscuring the true nature of mesmerism.

The literary representation of mesmerism in various genres, including novels, memoirs, biographies, detective stories, and horror stories, has profoundly ingrained itself in the Bengali psyche. However, the scarcity of authentic texts and the Bengali reluctance to engage with the subject have led to the emergence of unexplained and unscientific concepts. Prabhat Kumar Mukhopadhyay's *Shakha Vijay* (1881) exemplifies this trend, attempting to link mesmerism to non-scientific domains like tantra and magic. The text defines mesmerism as a hypnotic power to control another's soul, and describes its application as beginning with a special worship at the temple of Goddess Kamakhya. This conflation of scientific mesmerism with unscientific *vashikaran* (hypnotic control) marks a significant phase in the assimilation of mesmerism into unscientific territories, demonstrating the blurring of boundaries between science and pseudoscience in the Bengali imagination.

A plethora of literary works, including Damodara Mukhopadhyay's *Shukalbasona Sundari* (1884), Manoranjan Guha's *Asha Pradeep* (1889), and Saraladevi Chaudhurani's autobiographical work *Jibaner Jharapata* (1879), perpetuate the conflation of mesmerism with unscientific and pseudoscientific concepts. Saraladevi Chaudhurani's account of her neck pain being cured by H.S. Olcott sir through mesmerism and Navin Banerjee's depiction of his son's mesmerist abilities, alongside Shushila *bouthan*'s sudden and unexplained acquisition of mesmerist powers, exemplify this trend.[7] These works, which include accounts of mesmerism being used to cure ailments and grant unexplained powers, perpetuate a distorted understanding of the subject, leading to a diverse range of interpretations in the reader's mind. The lack of scientific explanation in these works contributes to the obfuscation of mesmerism's true nature, demonstrating the profound impact of literature on public understanding and perception. The lack of physical sensation experienced by patients during mesmerism and psychic treatments, as well as the comments made by psychic healers, spread among the Bengalis the idea that the doctor was in control of the patient's unconscious body, and the idea of seduction started to take hold among them at this point.

From Enigma to Enlightenment: The Resurgence of Mesmeric Healing in Modern Healthcare Education and Practice

In the twentieth century, British India continued to apply this paradigm, but eventually a new approach known as observational medicine arose. As a result, the focus of medicine has shifted from pathologic bodies to every single person in society. In order to demonstrate their rivalry for power Calcutta's aristocratic class vied with each other for domination of the Western hospitals. The British government required that this privilege for domination be exchanged for Rs 100 or 1000 *sicca* annually. This resulted in the appointment of Raja Buddhinath Roy, Raja Seebchunder, Nurshinghchunder Roy, Ram Comul Sen, Rustomjee Cowasji, and Dwarakanath Tagore as the hospital's administrators in Calcutta.[8] The prosperous financial situation of Calcutta's elites was utilised by Dr Edward, the principal of the Calcutta Medical College. One of the objectives was to develop Calcutta's medical market as a replacement for the industrial society in Britain because there was no tax levied on the import and export of British medicines in India. The Company then did not waste time in putting its newly acquired medical market into action through the Calcutta Medical College.[9] The medical field was first inspired by swadeshi or nationalist movements in the early twentieth century. The non-cooperation movement's supporters promoted Indian-origin medical systems instead of permitting the sick and underprivileged to use Western medical institutions. Nationalist groups responded strongly to the Medical Registration Acts of 1912 and 1914, which increased political pressure on the government.[10]

Bengal's influence on Indian politics started to wane with the annulment of the partition of Bengal in 1911, and the transfer of the capital from Bengal to Delhi. Additionally, due to Britain's direct involvement in the First World War, both crises were caused by British industrial and economic conditions. Between 1911 and 1921 there was economic turmoil, rising commodity prices, and escalating rates of unemployment. Domestic workers were engaged in labour work and earned a living at the time, while the educated middle class was in difficulties, for they were unable to perform any menial tasks, in their opinion. It became essential for the middle class to choose careers that required the absolute minimum amount of capital. For Calcutta's healthcare professionals, a brand-new occupation called a psychic healer was waiting for them in the second decade of the twentieth century. The educated middle class of Calcutta grasped the chance to operate in this field without a formal education or training. This helped to explain the enormous commercial success of psychic healing.[11]

Mesmerism and hypnotic application were said to be uncomplicated, rapid, and side-effect-free treatments for a wide range of complex illnesses. Such diseases included rheumatism, sleeplessness, menstrual irregularities, malaria, blindness, dyspepsia, hysteria, toothaches, paralysis, heart problems, mental illnesses, and many others.[12] The Western physicians of the day were likewise overwhelmed by this plethora of illnesses. Thus, Calcutta began to hear the names of a lot of psychic healers. Rajendra Rudra, the son of Kshitish Chandra Chakroborty, a Trataka Yoga specialist and psychical educator, was a well-known name among the psychic healers of this era. Particularly deserving of attention are Kunjabihari Bhattacharya, Surendra Mohan Bhattacharya, S.N. Bose, Dr N. Roy, and J. Choudhury.[13]

The preface of Prof. Rajendranath Rudra's book contains evidence of the public's desire for hypnotism and its study at this time. In all, he claimed to have hypnotised 16,000 persons while tutoring 400 others up to 1918.[14] The profession of psychic healers was becoming more and more commercialised. Psychic healers started selling various equipments used for treating illnesses. They even offered new users a fifty per cent price break on their course fees. Lessons in reading, meditation, hypnosis, and branch science cost sixty rupees each. Three shillings were enforced for its education by post in addition to practical education. One rupee and five rupees, respectively, were charged for personal letter clarification of doubts and personal demonstration at residence.[15]

Contrary to its historical association with pseudoscience, mesmerism has been revaluated and integrated into modern scientific practices, leveraging hypnosis and related techniques to address a range of physical and psychological health issues globally. The proliferation of academic programmes and courses in mesmerism, hypnotism, clinical hypnosis, and psychic healing across national and international institutions attests to the growing recognition of these modalities' therapeutic efficacy. This development marks a significant departure from mesmerism's earlier mystification, solidifying its legitimacy within the scientific community. The UGC Expert Committee on Model Psychology Courses for M.A. Specialization in Parapsychology has one such course. In this course, Paper I is on Historical Introduction to Parapsychology. A two-year Postgraduate Clinical Hypnosis programme is available at the University of Adelaide. The British College of Hypnosis & Hypnotherapy have introduced Post-graduate Diploma in Clinical Hypnosis. The M.S. University of Baroda, Vadodara have introduced Post Graduate Diploma in Clinical and Applied Hypnosis. Birmingham City University has also conducted a course of Clinical Hypnosis and Communication Techniques in Healthcare. Christ University has introduced a certificate course on clinical hypnosis. American Society for Clinical Hypnosis, Australian Society for Clinical Hypnosis, British Society of Clinical and Academic Hypnosis, National College of Hypnosis and Psychotherapy in UK, Clinical and Applied Hypnosis at Saybrook University in UK, and European Society of Hypnosis consist of forty-nine constituent societies in twenty-two countries throughout Europe. Clinical Hypnosis Training, at The Institute of Applied Psychology, Australia, is demonstrating daily that mesmerism and mesmeric treatments are not fiction but rather a method based on scientific truth. It will play a significant part in the healthcare institutions of the future because there are numerous other institutions where mesmerism is still practised.

It is now conceivable that mesmerism played a disruptive role in the nineteenth-century theatre of Calcutta's Western medical science. In the absence of chloroform, mesmerism was used to perform a number of painless operations. However, mesmerism and its first-generation implementers in Calcutta were swept away by the windfall of the Western market establishment. But if one looks at present times, one can identify that interest in the practice of hypnotism is gaining popularity worldwide. It appears that its implementation will proceed quickly in the field of general medicine. Overall, this study chronicles the earliest experience and voyage of anaesthetic surgery in nineteenth-century Calcutta.

While the chapters on imperialism and the numerous uprisings against it are the main draw of the modern historical context, a significant medical science breakthrough made after imperialism has remained out of the historical spotlight. In the study of surgery in India's history of medical practice in the later nineteenth century, mesmerism is still an intriguing concept. However, the need for extensive analytical research on the history of surgery in colonial Calcutta using this distinct treatment process has not seen much success. This research has revealed a crucial component of the history of surgery in colonial Bengal. It also strives to provide a detailed history of nineteenth-century Calcutta's distinctive pharmaceutical practices, as well as an examination of Calcutta's inhabitants in terms of their painless experience. The writing of this book serves as the preliminary step in the process of historically contextualising the importance of the mesmeric anaesthetic experience during surgical therapy in nineteenth-century Calcutta.

CONCLUSION

Mesmerism's Enduring Echoes in the Historical Symphony of Healing

In the captivating pages of nineteenth-century Calcutta's medical chronicle, the story of mesmerism unfolds like a spellbinding melody, where innovation, tradition and the quest for validation interweave to compose a symphony of healing. The expedition through this riveting journey has led us to the crossroads of mesmerism's enigmatic legacy, where its echoes reverberate through time, leaving an indelible mark on the evolution of medical science. Mesmerism, a remarkable healing method, encapsulated the promise of painless surgeries and transformative therapeutic experiences. Yet, its trajectory was far from linear, as the currents of societal change and the interplay between traditional wisdom and modern progress shaped its narrative. Calcutta, a vibrant hub of cultures, became the canvas upon which mesmerism's tale was painted, merging the alchemy of healing with the burgeoning innovations of Western medicine. The study of mesmerism presents a captivating exploration of the journey undertaken by mesmeric anaesthesia within the medical realm, with a particular focus on its application within the hospital in Calcutta. This tropical colony posed a formidable challenge for the British medical establishment due to its distinct environmental conditions. Concurrently, the introduction of packaged medicine marked a novel experience for the Bengali population.

The convergence of these factors set the stage for the dissemination and institutionalization of mesmeric practices within the healthcare framework, a seminal development that played a pivotal role in shaping the professionalization of healthcare and the broader medical culture in Bengal. Mesmerism, a practice attributed to Franz Mesmer, involved inducing a trance-like state in patients to alleviate pain and facilitate medical procedures. In the context of the hospital in Calcutta, this method gained prominence as an alternative approach to anaesthesia due to the efforts of Dr James Esdaile. The unique climate of the tropical colony presented its own set of challenges, demanding innovative solutions for effective healthcare delivery. Mesmeric anaesthesia emerged as an intriguing response to these challenges, offering a means to manage pain and discomfort in a resource-constrained environment. The introduction of packaged medicine added another layer to the evolving medical landscape in Bengal. This marked a departure from traditional herbal remedies and home-grown treatments, providing the Bengali populace access to standardized medicinal products. The juxtaposition of British medical practices and indigenous healing methods fostered a dynamic exchange of knowledge, shaping a hybrid medical culture that drew from diverse sources. As mesmeric anaesthesia gained acceptance, it not only transformed the patient experience but also prompted a shift towards a more systematic and structured approach to medical treatment. This transition marked a crucial step in the evolution of medical practices in Bengal, leading to the establishment of a more organized and regulated medical profession.

Furthermore, the infusion of mesmerism and packaged medicine into the healthcare fabric of Bengal also sparked discussions and debates around medical ethics and the cultural implications of these practices. The assimilation of these novel approaches raised questions about the balance between traditional healing wisdom and modern scientific methodologies, fostering a rich discourse that contributed to the maturation of medical thought in the region. The propagation and institutionalization of mesmeric practices extended beyond the confines of the hospital in Calcutta, permeating various strata of society. As the efficacy of mesmerism became more widely acknowledged, it garnered attention not only from the medical community but also from intellectuals, artists and the general public. This widespread interest sparked discussions and debates that contributed to the evolving medical discourse of the time. Moreover, the integration of mesmeric practices into medical education and training marked a transformative moment in the professionalization of healthcare, paving the way for a more structured and formalized medical curriculum in Bengal.

The exploration of mesmerism's journey within the medical field offers a captivating glimpse into the intricate interplay between scientific advancement, cultural exchange, and the aspirations of a burgeoning medical community. The hospital in Calcutta, situated at the crossroads of tradition and modernity, became a crucible for experimentation, where innovative approaches like mesmeric anaesthesia and packaged medicine catalysed a paradigm shift in medical practices. This transformative era laid the foundation for the evolution of a distinct medical identity in Bengal, one that continues to shape the region's healthcare landscape to this day. During the introduction of Western medicine and hospitalization to Bengal, the use of mesmerism for anaesthesia was a novel and unfamiliar application to the local population. Mesmerism, a technique involving inducing a trance-like state, was effectively utilized to alleviate body pain. However, it deviated from the conventional medicinal practices, as mesmerism didn't involve traditional medicines.

Western medicine sought to establish itself as a symbol of modernity and rational scientific methods, contrasting with the mystical and unconventional approach of mesmerism. Over time, Western medicine shifted its focus from *seva* (service) to a profit-oriented approach, viewing the diseased body as a lucrative market and healthcare as a capital-intensive enterprise.

Within this historical backdrop, Dr James Esdaile emerged as a visionary architect of change, crafting a legacy that would transcend time. His pioneering work in mesmeric anaesthesia and painless surgeries rewrote the conventions of medical practice, redefining the limits of human endurance and the realm of surgical possibilities. The Calcutta Mesmeric Hospital, a testament to his unwavering spirit, became a sanctuary where mesmerism's transformative potential was realized, offering a glimpse into the future of medical innovation.

However, the echoes of mesmerism's triumph were not immune to the shadows of ambivalence and eventual decline. The wavering support of Calcutta's elite, coupled with economic uncertainties, cast a veil of uncertainty over the Calcutta Mesmeric Hospital's legacy. The ascent of Western medicine, driven by imperialist fervour, marked a new chapter in medical history, signalling the twilight of mesmerism's influence in Bengal's healthcare landscape.

The tapestry of mesmerism's resonance extends beyond the confines of the nineteenth century, echoing through the corridors of time into our contemporary world. A glance through the lens of period newspapers and advertisements reveals the enduring impact of mesmerism, even in the face of evolving medical landscapes. Its legacy, though faded, endures as a testament to the pursuit of healing excellence, bridging eras and guiding the trajectory of medical progress.

In summation, our voyage through the captivating realm of mesmerism's narrative has illuminated the intricacies of a bygone era. This era, characterized by tradition, innovation, and the pursuit of Western validation, holds valuable insights for our understanding of medical history. As we bid farewell to the mesmerism of yesteryears, we embrace its legacy as a catalyst for change, a force that shaped the evolution of medicine, and a beacon that continues to illuminate the path toward healing in the intricate tapestry of time. The echoes of mesmerism's past resonate as a testament to human ingenuity, the unyielding spirit of progress, and the eternal quest to unravel the mysteries of healing in every chapter of history.

Endnotes

Introduction

1. Maris Loukas and Alexis Lanteri, "Anatomy in Ancient India: A Focus on the Susruta Samhita," *Journal of Anatomy*, Wiley Online Library, 217(6), 2010, pp. 646-650.
2. For details Anirban Banerjee and Anil Nanda, "Ambroise Paré and 16th Century Neurosurgery," *British Journal of Neurosurgery*, 25(2), 2011, pp. 193-196.
3. Jonathan Goddard, "Knife Man: The Extraordinary Life and Times of John Hunter, Father of Modern Surgery," *Journal of The Royal Society of London*, 98(7), 2005 July, p. 335.
4. Jacob Randolph, *A Memoir of the Life and Character of Philip Syng Physick*. Applewood's Medicine in America Series (Massachusetts, Philadelphia: Applewood Books, 1839), pp. 1-122.
5. R.J. Defalque and A.J. Wright, "The Short, Tragic Life of Robert M. Glover," *Anaesthesia*, 59, 2004, pp. 394–400.
6. William Hendrie, *Discovering West Lothian* (Edinburgh: John Donald, 1995), pp. 39-49.
7. Jonathan G. Hardman, *Oxford Textbook of Anaesthesia* (Oxford: Oxford University Press, 2017), p. 529.
8. Tyler Rouse, "A Brief and Strange History of Mesmerism and Surgery," *Hektoen International: A Journal of Medical Humanities*, 11(2) 2018, Tyler Rouse, Stratford.
9. George Sandby, *Mesmerism and its Opponents*, second edition (London: Longman, 1848), p. 52.
10. William Lang, *Animal Magnetism, or Mesmerism; Its History, Phenomena, and Present Condition: Containing Practical Instructions and The Latest Discoveries in The Science. Principally Derived From A Recent Work* (New York: James Mowatt & Co., 1844).
11. Catalın-Daniel Constantinescu and Lucian-Gabriel Petrescu, "Magnetic Materials, Thin Films and Nanostructures," *Magnetochemistry*, 9(5), May 2023, p. 133.
12. Lanto Thorvald Joks, "Scribonius Largus' Compounding of Drugs, Introduction, Translation, and Medico-Historical Comments," A PhD thesis submitted to the department of School of Humanities, Subject area Classics, College of Arts, University of Glasgow, June 2020, p. 165.

13 Stephen F. Keevil, "Physics and Medicine: a Historical Perspective," *Lancet* 2011; Vol. 379: 1519.

14 J. Lanska Douglas and T. Lanska Josep, "Franz Anton Mesmer and the Rise and Fall of Animal Magnetism: Dramatic Cures, Controversy, and Ultimately a Triumph for the Scientific Method," in *Brain, Mind and Medicine: Essays in Eighteenth-Century Neuroscience*, ed. Harry Whitaker, C.U.M. Smith, Stanley Finger (New York: Springer, 2007), pp. 301-320.

15 Robert Darnton, *Mesmerism and the End of the Enlightenment in France* (Cambridge: Harvard University Press, 1968), pp. 47-48.

16 Lang, *Animal Magnetism or Mesmerism*, p. 12.

17 Ibid., p. 55.

18 Baron Dupotet De Sennevoy, *An Introduction to the Study of Animal Magnetism* (London: Saunders & Otley, 1838), pp. 187-221.

19 Richard Chenevix, "On Mesmerism, Improperly denominated Animal Magnetism," *The London Medical and Physical Journal*, ed., John North and John Whatey, New Series, Vol. VI (London: Oxford University Press, 1829), pp. 219–230.

20 James Braid, *The Power of the Mind over the Body* (London: John Churchill, 1846), pp. 3-36.

21 Mary Elizabeth Leighton, "Hypnosis Redivivus": Ernest Hart, "British Medical Journal," and the Hypnotism Controversy, Victorian Periodicals Review The Johns Hopkins University Press on behalf of the Research Society for Victorian Periodicals, Summer, 2001, Vol. 34, No. 2, pp. 104-127.

22 Eric T. Carlson, "Charles Poyen Brings Mesmerism to America," *Journal of the History of Medicine and Allied Sciences*, 15(2) (Oxford University Press, 1960), pp. 121–32.

23 Sidney E. Lind, "Poe and Mesmerism," PMLA, vol. 62, no. 4 (Cambridge University Press, 1947), pp. 1077–94.

24 "Mott, Valentine," *Encyclopaedia Britannica* 18(11) (Cambridge University Press), p. 930.

25 John M. Carethers, "Diversification in the Medical Sciences Fuels Growth of Physician-Scientists," *The Journal of Clinical Investigation* 129(12), 2019, pp. 5051–54.

26 John Wakefield Francis, "Francis papers, 1789-1861," digitally accessed from Manuscripts and Archives Division, The New York Public Library.

27 Sandby, *Mesmerism and its Opponents*, p. 52.

28 A Summary of Persian Extracts From "Tabaqua-I-Mohsinj-A," A Persian History of the Imambarah written by Nawabzada Syed

Ashrafuddin Ahmed, Khan Bahadur, collected from the document *Collection Of Papers Relating To The Hooghly Imambarah 1815—1910* (Calcutta: Bengal Secretariat Book Depot, 1914).

29 *Report of the General Committee of Public Instruction (GCPI) of the Presidency of Fort William in Bengal for the year 1836* (Calcutta: The Baptist Mission Press, 1837).

30 Ramya Raman and A. Raman, "Painless Surgery Joseph Johnson Performed on a Mesmerized Patient in Madras in 1847," *Indian Journal of History of Science,* 54(1), 2019, pp. 13-22.

31 James Esdaile, *The Introduction of Mesmerism: As an Anaesthetic and Curative Agent into the Hospitals of India* (Perth, 1852).

32 G. Rosen, "Mesmerism and Surgery: A Strange Chapter in the History of Anaesthesia," *Journal of the History of Medicine and Allied Sciences,* 1(4), 1946, pp. 527-550.

33 "First Half-yearly Report of the Calcutta Mesmeric Hospital. From 1st September, 1848, to 1st March, 1849," *The Zoist,* XXVI, July 1849, p. 129.

34 See Joseph Ennemoser, *The History of Magic,* trans., William Howitt, vol I (London, 1854), p. 392.

35 Waltraud Ernst, "'Under the Influence' in British India: James Esdaile's Mesmeric Hospital in Calcutta, and its Critics," *Psychological Medicine,* 25 (Cambridge: Cambridge University Press, 1995), pp. 1113-1123.

36 Srilata Chatterjee, *Western Medicine and Colonial Society: Hospitals of Calcutta, c. 1757 – 1860* (Delhi: Primus Books, 2017), p. 217.

37 "The Protest and Petition to James Esdaile, Surgeon, H.E.I.C.S", collected from the journal *The Zoist: A Journal of Cerebral Physiology and Mesmerism and their Application to Human Welfare,* Vol. II, March 1853 to January 1854 (London: Hippolyte Bailliere Press), pp. 294-297.

38 Lindsay B. Yeates, "James Braid: Chemical and Hypnotic Anaesthesia, Psycho-Physiology, and Braid's Final Theories," *Australian Journal of Clinical Hypnotherapy and Hypnosis,* 40(2), Spring 2018, p. 112.

39 J.F. Clarke, "A Strange Chapter in the History of Medicine," in *Autobiographical Recollections of the Medical Profession* (London: J & A Churchill, 1874), pp. 155-169.

Journey of Western Medicine in Nineteenth-Century Calcutta

1 Pratik Chakrabarti, *Medicine and Empire, 1600-1960* (New York: Palgrave Macmillan, 2014), pp. 41-43.

2 Ives Edward, *Voyage from the England to India in the year MDCCLIV (1754) and an Historical Narrative of The Operation of the Squadron*

and Army in India, Under the Command of Vice-Admiral Watson and Colonel Clive, in the Years 1755, 1756, 1757; including a Correspondence between the Admiral and the Nabob Serajah Dowlah (London: Edward and Charles Dilly, 1774), pp. 89-187.

3 Ibid., p. 448.

4 Chatterjee, *Western Medicine and Colonial Society*, p. 70.

5 Omkar Goswami, "Sahibs, Babus, and Banias: Changes in Industrial Control in Eastern India, 1918-50," *The Journal of Asian Studies*, 48(2), May 1989, pp. 289-309.

6 Nandini Bhattacharya, *Disparate Remedies: Making Medicines in Modern India* (McGill-Queen's University Press, 2023), pp. 33-36.

7 Jadunath Sarkar, *History of Bengal* vol. 2 (Dhaka University, 1948), p. 379.

8 Anjali Basu, "Bengal in the Reign of Aurangzib (1658-1707)," Thesis submitted at the University of London, School of Oriental and African Studies (London: 1965), pp. 177-250.

9 G. Jan Meulenbeld and Wujastyk Domin, *Studies on Indian Medical History* vol. V (Delhi: Motilal Banarsidass Publications, 2001), pp. 27-29.

10 Subodh Kant Pandey, Mahendrasing Patil and Swapnil Raskar, "Kashyapa Samhita: A Review of History & Its Contribution to Kaumarbhritya," in *European Journal of Biomedical and Pharmaceutical Sciences*, Vol. 6(5), 2019: pp. 640-644.

11 P.K.J.P. Subhaktha, "Cakrapénidatta" in *Bulletin of the Indian Institute of History of Medicine* vols 22–23 (Indian Institute of History of Medicine, 1992), p. 53.

12 W.H.S. Jones ed. and trans., *Hippocrates Collected Works I* (Cambridge: Harvard University Press, 1868), p. 11.

13 Ibid., pp. 116-130.

14 H.E. Sigerist, *A History of Medicine*, vol. III (New York: Oxford University Press, 1961), pp. 137-148.

15 S.N. Sen, "A Survey of Source Material," in D.M. Bose ed., *A Concise History of Science in India* (New Delhi: Indian National Science Academy, 1971), p. 16.

16 B.L. Gordon, *Medicine Throughout Antiquity* (Philadelphia: F.A. Davis Company, 1949), pp. 313–317.

17 D.P. Chattopadhyay, *What is Living and What is Dead in Indian Philosophy* (New Delhi: People's Publishing House, 1976), p. 236.

18 C.K. Gamage, "Dissemination of Knowledge for Health and Wellbeing: with Special Reference to Buddhism and Ayurveda,"

Sri Lanka Journal of Indigenous Medicine, Institute of Indigenous Medicine 7(2), 2022: pp. 658-66.

19 J. Bhattacharya, "The Hospital Transcends into Hospital Medicine: A Brief Journey through Ancient, Medieval and Colonial India," in *Indian Journal of History of Science* 52(1), 2017, pp. 28-53.

20 Radha Kumud Mookherji, *The Gupta Empire* (Delhi: Motilal Banarsidass Publications, 1989), p. 61.

21 Sigerist, *A History of Medicine*, pp. 137-48.

22 Pasha M. Azeez, *Maden-Ush-Shifa Tibbe Sikender Shahi*. Compiled in the time of Sultan Sikender Shah Lodi (1488-1518) by his courtier, Behwa bin Qewas Khan. It also contains the summary of 13 Ayurvedic books then existing in India. Chapter 1 Section IX, "Preservation of Health and Prevention of Diseases," *Bulletin of the Institute of History of Medicine*, Hyderabad 2(1), 1972, pp. 17-22.

23 Trihumoral theory is the core of Ayurveda. In the living, there are only three fundamental mechanisms happening at all times. One mechanism is known as catabolism: breaking down the food or tissue to provide energy. The other mechanism which is called anabolism utilizes this energy to facilitate growth and repair. The third mechanism is an entity which strives to maintain a balance between these two.

24 Mohammad Habib Khalid Ahmad Nizam, *A Comprehensive History of India*, vol. 5: *The Delhi Sultanate (A.D. 1206-1526)* (Delhi: People's Publishing House, 1970), p. 604.

25 Ibid., p. 924.

26 M.Z. Siddiqui, "The Unani-Tibb (Greek Medicine) in India," in D.M. Bose ed. *Concise History*, p. 272.

27 Nadeem Rezavi and S. Ali, "Physicians as Professionals in Medieval India," in Deepak Kumar ed. *Disease and Medicine in India* (Delhi: Tulika Books, 2012), pp. 40-65.

28 R.L. Verma and N.H. Keswani, "Unani Medicine in Medieval India: Its Teachers and Texts" in N.H. Keswani ed. *The Science of Medicine and Physiological Concepts in Ancient and Medieval India* (New Delhi: S.K. Manchanda, 1974), p. 137.

29 J. Bhattacharya, "The Hospital Transcends into Hospital Medicine: A Brief Journey through Ancient, Medieval and Colonial India," *Indian Journal of History of Science* 52(1), 2017, pp. 31-37.

30 D. Kumar, "Adoption and Adaption: A Study of Medical Ideas and Techniques in Colonial India," in F. Günergun and D. Raina ed. *Science between Europe and Asia: Boston Studies in the Philosophy of Science* 275 (2017): pp. 233-45.

31 S. Mukherjee, "Medicine and Public Health in Modern Bengal

1850-1950," in S. Bhattacharya ed. *A Comprehensive History of Modern Bengal 1700–1950* vol. 2 (Kolkata: The Asiatic Society, 2020), pp. 702-703.

32 Alexander Hamilton, *A New Account of The East Indies, With Numerous Maps & Illustrations edited with Introduction and Notes by Sir William Foster*, vol. II (London: The Argonaut Press, 1930), p. 174.

33 Ibid., p. 7.

34 D. Arnold, *The New Cambridge History of India, Science Technology and Medicine in Colonial India*, 3(5), (Cambridge University Press, 2020), pp. 58-59.

35 Bhattacharya (2017), p. 40.

36 M. Harrison, "Racial Pathologies: Morbid Anatomy in British India, 1770–1850," in B. Pati & M. Harrison ed. *The Social History of Health and Medicine in Colonial India* (London: Routledge, 2009), pp. 173-194.

37 D. Kumar, "Science in Modern Bengal," in S. Bhattacharya ed. *A Comprehensive History of Modern Bengal 1700 – 1950* vol. 3 (Kolkata: The Asiatic Society, 2020), pp. 491-537.

38 D. Arnold, *Colonizing the Body: State Medicine and Epidemic Disease in Nineteenth Century India* (California: University of California Press, 1993), pp. 49 –58.

39 Bhattacharya (2017), p. 45.

40 Anshu and A. Supe, "Evolution of Medical Education in India: The Impact of Colonialism," *Journal of Postgraduate Medicine*, 62(4), 2016, pp. 255-259.

41 Ibid.

42 D. Arnold (2000), pp. 61-70.

43 Samita Sen and Anirban Das, "History of the Calcutta Medical College and Hospital, 1835 - 1936," in *History of Science, Philosophy and Culture in Indian Civilization*, General Editor, D.P. Chattopadhyaya, Volume XV, Part 4, *Science and Modern India: An Institutional History, c.1784-1947*, ed. Uma Das Gupta (Delhi: Pearson Education Publication, Centre for Studies in Civilization, 2011), pp. 477-522.

44 Bhattacharya (2017), pp. 47–48.

45 C. Hochmuth, "Patterns of Medical Culture in Colonial Bengal, 1835 –1880," *Oxford Bulletin of the History of Medicine* 81(1), 2006, pp. 39-72.

46 "Annual Report of the Medical College of Bengal Twelfth Year – 1846," *Calcutta Review* 7, January to June 1847, Xlii – Xlix. See – Anonymous.

47 S. Mukherjee (2020), p. 699.

48 R. Jeffery, "Recognizing India's doctors: The Institutionalization of Medical Dependency, 1918–1939," *Modern Asian Studies* 13 (1979): 301–26.
49 Hochmuth (2006), p. 57.
50 C. Palit & T. Goswami, "Sanitation, Empire, Environment: Bengal (1880 –1920)," *Proceedings of the Indian History Congress* 68 (2007): 731–44.
51 P.B. Mukherjee, "Pharmacology, 'Indigenous knowledge', Nationalism," in B. Pati & M. Harrison ed. *The Social History of Health and Medicine in Colonial India* (London: Routledge, 2009), p. 198.
52 Sutapa Dutta, "Packing a Punch at the Bengali Babu," *South Asia Journal of South Asian Studies* (Routledge, 2021), pp.1-22.

Mesmeric Anaesthetic Surgeries at the Calcutta Mesmeric Hospital

1 James Esdaile, *Mesmerism in India and its Practical Application in Surgery and Medicine* (London: Longman, 1846), pp. 1-2.
2 *The Zoist: A Journal of Cerebral Physiology and Mesmerism and their Application to Human Welfare*, vol. IX, March 1851 to January 1852 (London: Hippolyte Bailliere Press, 1852), p. 93.
3 D.J. Lanska, J.T. Lanska, "Franz Anton Mesmer and the Rise and fall of Animal Magnetism: Dramatic Cures, Controversy, and Ultimately a Triumph for the Scientific Method," in H. Whitaker, C.U.M. Smith, S. Finger, eds *Brain, Mind and Medicine: Essays in Eighteenth-Century Neuroscience* (2017), pp. 23-30.
4 Ivan P. Pavlov, *Psychopathology and Psychiatry* (USA: Transaction Publication, 1994), pp. 408–26.
5 Frank Podmore (1909), pp. 61-101.
6 Esdaile (1846), pp. 96-97.
7 F.A. Pattie, "Mesmer's Medical Dissertation and its Debt to Mead's De Imperio Solis ac Lunae," *Journal of History of Medicine and Allied Science* 11(3), 1956, pp. 275-87.
8 Richard Harte, *Hypnotism and The Doctors. Vol I. Animal Magnetism. Mesmer: His Theory of Disease. His Method of Cure. His Fight with the Faculty. De Puysegur: Somnambulism. New Theories and Methods.* (London: L. N. Fowler & Co., 1902), pp. 14-15.
9 S. Stubner and Schulz, "Clinical Hypnosis and Anaesthesia: An Historical Review and Its Clinical Implications in Today's Practice," *Bulletin Anesthesia History* 18(1), 2000, pp. 4-5.
10 Benjamin Franklin, "The Reports of the Royal Commission of 1784 on Mesmer's System of Animal Magnetism and Other

Contemporary Documents, 11 August 1784." Translated by I.M.L. Donaldson. Published for the James Lind Library, Sibbald Library and Royal College of Physicians of Edinburgh (Edinburgh, 2014), p. 21.

11 Mary Elizabeth Leighton, "Hypnosis Redivivus": Ernest Hart, "British Medical Journal", and the Hypnotism Controversy, *Victorian Periodicals Review The Johns Hopkins University Press on behalf of the Research Society for Victorian Periodicals,* 34(2), 2001, pp. 104-107.

12 Stubner, S. Schulz, op. cit., pp. 22-28.

13 Richard Chenevix, "On Mesmerism, improperly denominated Animal Magnetism," *The London Medical and Physical Journal* (ed.) John North, John Whatey, New Series, Vol. VI (London: Oxford University Press, 1829), pp. 219–230.

14 Chenevix, op. cit., pp. 229–230.

15 George Rosen, "John Elliotson Physician and Hypnotist," in *Bulletin of the Institute of the History of Medicine,* 4(7), 1936, pp. 600–03.

16 E.S. Ridgway, "John Elliotson (1791–1868): A Bitter Enemy of Legitimate Medicine? Part I: Earlier Years and the Introduction to Mesmerism," in *Journal of Medical Biography,* 1(4), 1993: 191-198.

17 C.D. James, "Mesmerism: A Prelude to Anaesthesia," *A Proceeding of The Royal Society of Medicine,* 68(7), 1975, pp. 446-447.

18 C.A. Fuge, "Bedford Square: A Connexion with Mesmerism," 41(7), 1986, pp. 726-730.

19 Waltraud Ernst, "'Under the influence' in British India: James Esdaile's Mesmeric Hospital in Calcutta, and its Critics," *Psychological Medicine,* 25 (6), 1995, pp. 13-112.

20 See *The Asiatic Journal and Monthly Register for British and Foreign India, China, Australia,* Vol–XVIII, New Series (W.M.H. Allen, 1835), p. 241.

21 James Esdaile, *Mesmerism in India and its Practical Application in Surgery and Medicine* (New York: Silas Andrus and Son, 1851), pp. 61-65.

22 James Esdaile had been reading about the mesmeric anaesthesia experiments from various books and journals between 1839 to 1841 including *The Zoist* by Dr Elliotson, *Facts in Mesmerism with Reasons for a Dispassionate Inquiry into it* (1839) by Rev. Chauncey Hare Townshend, and *Introduction Au Magnetism* (1840) by M. Aubin Gautier.

23 It is the deepest stage of Hypnosis. Hypnotic suggestions that are given in this state become convictions automatically because the subject does not remember them. It is a state of deep sleep, where the

mesmerised person may respond with amnesia, anaesthesia, negative or positive hallucinations, and the complete control of senses.

24 Esdaile, 1950, op. cit., p. 76.
25 Ibid., pp. 79-80.
26 Ibid., pp. 190-191.
27 A wooden framework, sometimes with cloth extensions, hung from the ceiling with an attachment of rope/wire which was pulled at the other end by a human operator.
28 Esdaile 1846, op. cit., pp. 204-205.
29 Esdaile 1850, op. cit., p. 80.
30 Ibid., pp. 65-66.
31 Ibid., pp. 192-193.
32 Ibid., p. 193.
33 Ibid., pp. 194-195.
34 Ibid., pp. 72, 124.
35 Ibid., pp. 168-170.
36 Ibid., pp. 195-196.
37 Ibid., p. 196.
38 Ibid., pp. 146-149.
39 Ibid., pp. 173-174.
40 Ibid., pp. 94-95.
41 Ibid., p. 197.
42 Ibid., p. 105.
43 Ibid., pp. 201-202.
44 Ibid., p. 202.
45 Ibid., pp. 150-151.
46 Ibid., pp. 220-244.
47 Source: Esdaile, *Mesmerism in India and Its Practical Application*, p. XVIII. Also, to know the individual names of patients please see pp. 143-210.
48 Elliotson, *The Zoist,* vol – IV, pp. 193-194.
49 Ibid., p. 195.
50 To know more about these cases see Elliotson, *The Zoist,* vol. IV, pp. 286-290.
51 A. Sylvain Lee, *The Practice of Hypnotic Suggestion* (United States: Missouri Institution of Science, 1901), p. 11.

52 Jackson J. Howard, Frederick Arthur, ed., *Visitation of England and Wales*, Vol. 5 (Priv. Printed, London: 1897), p. 28.

53 *The Original Report of The Committee Appointed by Government to Observe and Report upon Surgical Operation by Dr. J. Esdaile, Upon Patients under the Influence of Alleged Mesmeric Agency* (Calcutta: Military Orphan Press, 1846). Wood Library Museum of Anaesthesiology. 1061 American Lane, Schaumburg, USA, American Society of Anaesthesiology.

54 *Dr. Stewart's Notes of Dr. Esdaile's Mesmeric Operation on the 14th October. Original Report of Mesmeric Committee, 1846*, p. 27.

55 To read the detailed original report see Appendix 13 A & B.

56 Ibid., p. 29.

57 Ibid.

58 *The Calcutta Star,* 15th October, 1846.

59 *Ceylon Observer,* 19th November, 1846.

60 *Delhi Gazette,* 24th December, 1846.

61 Elliotson, *The Zoist* vol. VI, pp. 10-12.

62 Ibid., pp.13-17.

63 Ibid., pp. 17-18.

64 Ibid., p. 18.

65 Ibid., pp. 18-19.

66 Ibid., p. 21.

67 Ibid., pp. 22-23.

68 Ibid., p. 27.

69 Ibid., p. 32.

70 Ibid., pp. 33-34.

71 Ibid., pp. 35-36.

72 Ibid., p. 36.

73 Ibid, pp. 38-39.

74 Ibid., pp. 39-40.

75 *Bengal and Agra (Miscellaneous), The Indian News, The Indian News and Chronicle of Eastern Affairs,* London, 5th January 1849, p. 481.

76 *Record of Cases Treated in the Mesmeric Hospital; From June To December 1847, 1848,* op. cit., pp. 3-4.

77 Ibid., pp. 10-11.

78 Ibid., p. 75.

79 Ibid., p. 79.

Endnotes

80   Elliotson, *The Zoist*, pp. 19-21.
81   Ibid, p. 20.
82   Ibid., pp. 23-24.
83   *Record of Cases Treated in the Mesmeric Hospital; From June To December 1847,* op. cit., pp. 39-49.
84   Ibid., pp. 32-33.
85   Elliotson, *The Zoist*, pp. 34-35.
86   Ibid., p. 39.
87   Ibid., p. 41.
88   *Record of Cases Treated in the Mesmeric Hospital; From June To December 1847,* op. cit., p. 2.
89   Ibid., p. 11.
90   Ibid., pp. 11-12.
91   Ibid., p. 21.
92   Ibid., pp. 59-61.
93   Ibid., pp. 61-62.
94   Ibid., pp. 71-72.
95   Ibid., pp. 72-73.
96   Ibid., pp. 73-74.
97   Ibid., p. 75.
98   Ibid., p. 84.
99   Elliotson, *The Zoist*, pp. 30-31.
100 Ibid., pp. 31-32.
101 Ibid., p. 31.
102 Ibid.
103 *All the Report of Return of Surgical Operations Performed In The Calcutta Mesmeric Hospital, From November 1846 To 1st January 1848, has been collected from The Original Report of Record of Cases Treated In The Mesmeric Hospital From June To December 1847; With Reports Of The Official Visitors,* Printed By Order Of Government, Calcutta, W. Ridsdale, Military Orphan Press, 1848. pp. 104-111. An author collection from Yale Medical Library, Historical Library Section
104 To read the report of Lord Dalhousie see Appendix 4.
105 Elliotson, *The Zoist* vol. VI, p. 114.
106 Ibid., p. 120.

Exploring the Final Phase of Mesmerism

1. Elliotson, *The Zoist*, p. 70.
2. James Esdaile, *Natural and Mesmeric Clairvoyance with the Practical Application of Mesmerism in Surgery and Medicine* (London: Hippolyte Bailliere, 1852), p. 2.
3. D.G. Crawford, *A History of The Indian Medical Service 1600-1913*, Volume II (London: Thacker Spink & Co., 1914), p. 155.
4. "Triumph and Reward of Dr. Esdaile," *The Zoist*, vol xxii, July 1848, p. 116.
5. Ibid., p. 114.
6. Elliotson, *The Zoist* vol. VI, p. 166.
7. Ibid., vol. V, p. 413.
8. Ibid., p. 150.
9. Ibid., vol. VI, p. 161.
10. Ibid., vol. IV, p. 576.
11. "Mesmeric Hospital; To The Right Hon. The Earl of Dalhousie, Triumph and Reward of Dr. Esdaile," in *The Zoist*, vol. Xxii, 1848, p. 119.
12. Elliotson, *The Zoist* vol. VI, p. 396.
13. James Esdaile, *The Introduction of Mesmerism as an Anesthetic and Curative Agent in to the Hospital of India* (Perth, 1852), pp. 18-29.
14. Elliotson, *The Zoist* vol. VI, p. 395.
15. Chatterjee, *Western Medicine and Colonial Society*, p. 217.
16. John Elliotson, *Mesmerism in India, Second Half Yearly Report of the Calcutta Mesmeric Hospital, From 1st March to 1st September, 1849*, 2nd edition (London: Hippolyte Bailliere, 1849), pp. 3-11.
17. Elliotson, *The Zoist* vol. Vii, pp. 124-126.
18. Ibid., pp. 126-127.
19. Ibid., p. 134.
20. Ibid., p. 121.
21. Elliotson, *Mesmerism in India*, op. cit., p. 7.
22. Blair B. Kling, "Chapter IX. The fall of the union bank," in *Partner in Empire: Dwarkanath Tagore and the Age of Enterprise in Eastern India* (Berkeley: University of California Press, 1976), pp. 198-229.
23. Elliotson, *The Zoist* vol. VI, pp. 396-97.
24. See "Medical Appointment, Bengal," in *Allen's Indian Mail and Register of Intelligence for British and Foreign India, China, and All*

Part of *The East,* Vol IX, January to June 1851 (London: W.M.H. Allen and Co.), p. 292.

25 "An Account of the Mesmeric Hospital in Bengal since Dr. Esdaile's departure from India," *The Zoist* vol. 10, no. 39 (October 1852), p. 281.

26 D.H. Robinson and A.H. Toledo, "Historical Development of Modern Anaesthesia," *Journal of Investigative Surgery; The official Journal of The Academy of Surgical Research,* 25(3), 2012, pp. 141-9.

27 Patrick Hehir, "The Hyderabad Chloroform Commissions," *Indian Medical Gazette,* April 1893, pp. 103-106.

28 E. Lawrie, *Report of the Hyderabad Chloroform Commission* (Bombay: Printed at the Times of India Steam Press, 1891), pp. 5-7.

29 M.H. Armstrong Davison, "Chloroform," *British Journal of Anaesthesia* (England: Oxford Publishing Limited, 1965), p. 656.

30 D.G. Tendulkar, *Mahatma Gandhi* vol. 2, (Publications Division, Ministry of Information and Broadcasting, Government of India, 1969), p. 76.

31 *Mesmerism In The East: Communicated By Dr. Elliotson, Report of the Calcutta Mesmeric Hospital for October.* By James Esdaile, M.D., Presidency Surgeon. From the Indian Reporter of Medical Science.

32 Elliotson, *Mesmerism in India; Second Half Yearly Report of The Calcutta Mesmeric Hospital From 1st March to 1st September 1849,* pp. 122-123.

33 Ibid., pp. 4-5.

34 Poonam Bala, *Imperialism and Medicine in Bengal* (New Delhi: Sage Publications, 1991), p. 78.

35 Ishita Pande, *Medicine, Race and Liberalism in British Bengal* (London: Routledge, 2010), pp. 277-279.

36 Sarmistha De, "Dominating the Body and Mind: Calcutta Medical College," in *Calcutta in the Nineteenth Century,* ed, Bidisha Chakraborty and Sarmistha De (New Delhi: Niyogi Books, 2014), pp. 307-308.

37 Esdaile, *Mesmerism in India and Its Practical Application,* p. 15.

38 Esdaile, "Mesmerism in the East", in *The Zoist,* ed John Elliotson, vol. VII, March 1849 – January 1850, pp. 121-137.

39 Ernst, "'Under the influence' in British India", pp. 1113-1123.

40 Esdaile, *Mesmerism in India and its Practical Application in Surgery and Medicine,* p. 43.

41 Chatterjee, *Western Medicine and Colonial Society,* p. 272.

42 Anindita Mukhopadhyay, "The Making of the Mask, 1854–90,"

Behind the Mask: The Cultural Definition of the Legal Subject in Colonial Bengal 1715-1911 (Delhi: 2006; online edition, Oxford Academic, 18 Oct. 2012).

43   *Dr Thomson's report from The Visitor to Calcutta Mesmeric Hospital,* Medical Board Proceeding, July–August 1847.

44   *Report of Dr. J. Mouat, Medical College, 9th December 1847, Record of Cases Treated in the Mesmeric Hospital; From June To December 1847,* Printed by Order of Government (Calcutta: Military Orphan Press, 1848).

45   Ibid., p. xliii

46   Ibid., pp. h to li.

Mesmerism's Legacies

1   Bala, *Imperialism and Medicine in Bengal,* p. 75.

2   Annie Besant, *The Ancient Wisdom: An Outline of Theosophical Teachings* (Adyar, Madras: Theosophical Publishing House, 1919), p. 1.

3   Shreya Chakravorty, "Swarnakumari Devi and Mesmerism," Academia: Basanti Devi College, 4(3), 2023, pp. 104-113.

4   "The Theosophist: A Monthly Journal Devoted to Oriental Philosophy, Art, Literature And Occultism: Embracing Mesmerism, Spiritualism, And Other Secret Sciences," IV, Suppl. to April, 1883, (On 30th March 1883, ODL., II, 411), p. 6.

5   Brojendranath Bandyopadhyay, "*Jantob Chumbak-Shakti,*" ed, Swarnakumari Devi, *Bharati, Magh* 1300 (Jan-Feb 1894), pp. 632-635.

6   Prabhat Kumar Mukhopadhyay, "*Jogobal na Psychic Force,*" in *Golpo Samagra,* vol. 4, p. 68.

7   Saraladevi Choudhurani, *Jibaner Jharapata* (Sahitya Sangsad, 1879), pp. 57-58.

8   Chatterjee, *Western Medicine and Colonial Society,* p. 145.

9   Bala, op. cit., p. 67.

10   Ibid., pp. 88-89.

11   Runa Das Choudhury, op. cit., pp. 86–103.

12   Ibid.

13   Ibid., p. 89.

14   Rajendranath Rudra, *Sammohan Vidya,* 4th edition (Calcutta: printed by Kalachand Basak, Narayan Machine Press, 1935), p. 13.

15   Ibid., Annexes.

APPENDICES

Appendix 1

Report of the Mesmeric Committee appointed by the Government to observe and report upon surgical operations by James Esdaile.

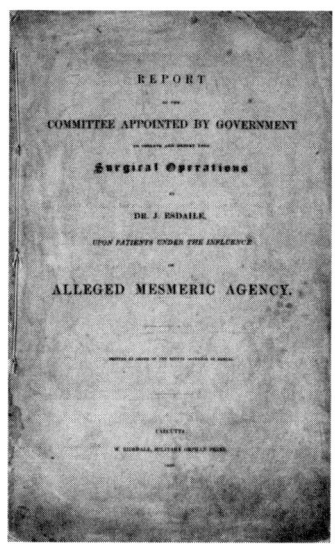

Source: *The Original Report of The Committee Appointed by Government to Observe and Report upon Surgical Operation by Dr. J. Esdaile, Upon Patients Under The Influence of Alleged Mesmeric Agency*, Military Orphan Press, Calcutta, 1846. Collected from Wood Library Museum of Anesthesiology, Front Page.

Appendix 2

Dr Jackson's Report on Mesmeric Surgery by Dr J. Esdaile

DR. JACKSON'S REPORT.

FROM J. JACKSON, ESQ.,
Surgeon to the Native Hospital,
TO J. FORSYTH, ESQ.,
Secretary to the Medical Board,
Fort William.

SIR,

A year having passed since the establishment of the Experimental Mesmeric Hospital, I have now, as one of the visitors appointed by Government, and in obedience to their orders, the honor of transmitting to the Medical Board, my report on what I have witnessed.

I have also the honor of forwarding at the same time a statement of the number and result of the operations which have taken place during the last year in the Hospital I have charge of, which the Government have called for at the suggestion of Dr. Esdaile, in order that a comparison may be made between their results, and those performed by Dr. Esdaile, under the Mesmeric Agency.

I have, &c.,
(Signed) J. JACKSON,
Surgeon to the Native Hospital.

Native Hospital, Nov. 22d, 1847.

FROM DR. JACKSON,
Visitor Mesmeric Hospital,
TO THE SECRETARY MEDICAL BOARD,
Dated 16th November, 1847.

SIR,

Since the establishment of the Mesmeric Hospital I have been a frequent visitor, and have witnessed several operations performed by Dr. Esdaile whilst the patients were in a mesmeric state, but in none have I observed any feature differing from the account given in the original Report of the Mesmeric Committee, of which I was a Member in the latter part of last year.

Hindoos, suffering from hypertrophy of the scrotum, with which they had been afflicted for years, were for the most part, the class operated on: the time required to bring them under the mesmeric state was generally from five to fifteen days, some few were brought under the influence at an earlier period, whilst others were

Source: *Record of Cases Treated in the Mesmeric Hospital; From June To December 1847,* Printed by Order of Government, Military Orphan Press, Calcutta, 1848.

Appendix 3

Dr James Esdaile's Experimental Report on Mesmeric Surgery from Dr O'Shaughnessy, Professor of Surgery, Calcutta Medical College

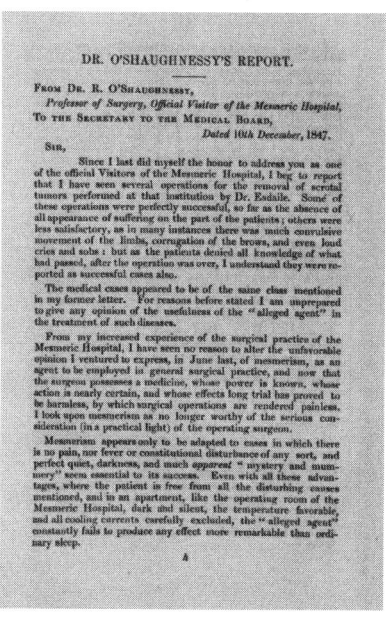

Plate - A

Source: *Record of Cases Treated in the Mesmeric Hospital; From June To December 1847,* Printed by Order of Government, Military Orphan Press, Calcutta, 1848. p. H.

> Except the occasional production of insensibility, which it can no longer claim the exclusive power of effecting, I saw no advantage, either to the patient or the surgeon, which could be fairly attributed to mesmerism. The haemorrhage was as severe as is usual in such operations. The nature of the operation was in no instance modified, so as to improve the ultimate condition of the patient. The ease, coolness, and deliberation of the surgeon did not appear to me to be at all increased, by the apparently unconscious state of his patients; nor were the slow dissections, sometimes necessary for the purpose of preserving important parts, had recourse to more frequently, or indeed so frequently with success, as I have seen in other hospitals; on the contrary, the dread that the patient might wake up, and spoil the experiment before the operation was concluded, appeared to me, to act most injuriously on the nerves of the operator, and to produce a hurry, and want of precision in his proceedings, most unfavourable both to himself and to his patients.
>
> Contrast this with the newly discovered agent, ether. It is equally efficacious, and certain in its effects, when administered to a patient writhing in agony from a recent wound, or about to undergo an operation for a painless tumour. It may be employed with equal success in the most noisy as in the most silent situations, and therefore it is available for the most urgent cases, and for Military, as well as for Civil Surgery. I have employed this agent in every surgical case of the least importance requiring operation, both in private and hospital practice, for the last nine months, with the most satisfactory results. At first I occasionally failed to produce perfect insensibility with it, owing to bad ether, imperfect apparatus, and the timidity of ignorance (for I dreaded to use, as freely as I might, a power of so apparently formidable a nature); but I now find that in every instance it produces perfect insensibility, which may be kept up, or allowed to pass away, at pleasure, and I have not in a single instance had cause to regret its employment.
>
> I feel that I should apologise for offering my opinion of the use of ether, in a report upon Mesmerism as practised under Dr. Esdaile; but as that gentleman took much unnecessary trouble (which no doubt was disinterested and well meant) both in the newspapers, and in his official correspondence, to prejudice the public and the profession against its use, I feel it to be my duty to state the result of my experience of this inestimable boon, with the hope of counteracting, as much as my humble opinion may tend to do so, the prejudice and alarm attempted to be created against it.

Plate - B

Source: *Record of Cases Treated in the Mesmeric Hospital; From June To December 1847,* Printed by Order of Government, Military Orphan Press, Calcutta, 1848. p. L.

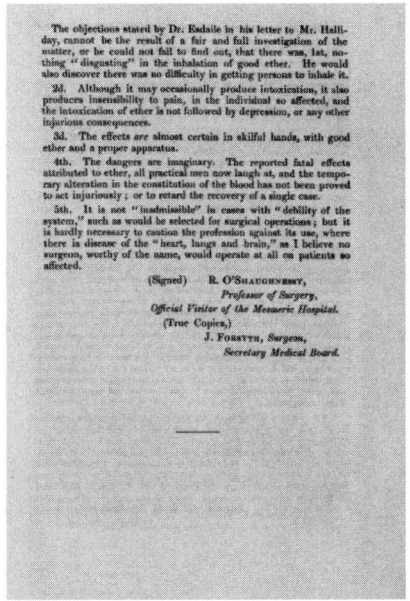

Plate - C

Source: *Record of Cases Treated in the Mesmeric Hospital; From June To December 1847, Printed by Order of Government,* Military Orphan Press, Calcutta, 1848. p. li.

Appendix 4

Letter from the Marquis of Dalhousie on Mesmeric Surgery by Dr James Esdaile

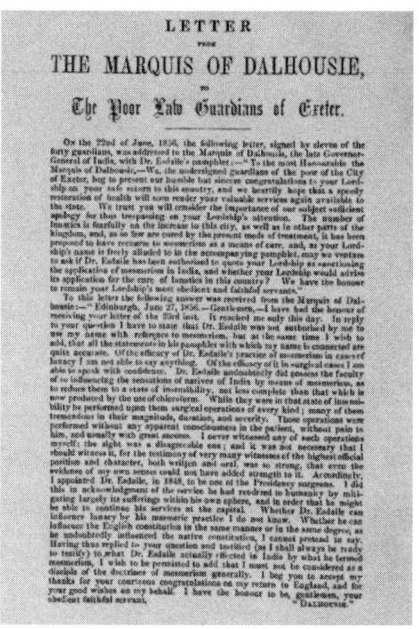

Source: *The Introduction of Mesmerism (with the Sanction of the Government) Into the Public Hospitals of India* by James Esdaile, M.D. Second Edition. W. Kent & Co. London, 1856, p. 1.

Appendix 5

A sketch of the patient Kanho with his tumour who was cured through mesmeric anaesthesia by Dr James Esdaile

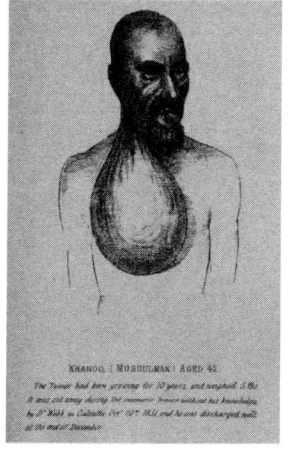

Source: *The Introduction of Mesmerism (with the Sanction of the Government) Into the Public Hospitals of India* by James Esdaile, M.D. Second Edition. W. Kent & Co. London, 1856.

Appendix 6

A sketch of a tumour of the antrum maxillare treated by James Esdaile through mesmeric anaesthetic surgery

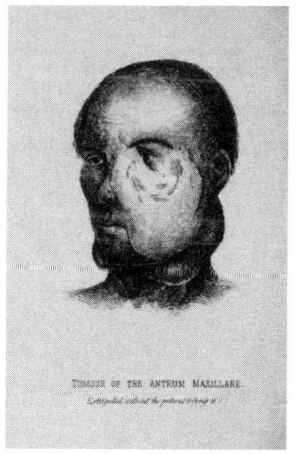

Source: *The Introduction of Mesmerism (with the Sanction of the Government) Into the Public Hospitals of India* by James Esdaile, M.D. Second Edition. W. Kent & Co. London, 1856.

Appendix 7

A sketch of mesmeric sleep before the operation of breast tumour by James Esdaile

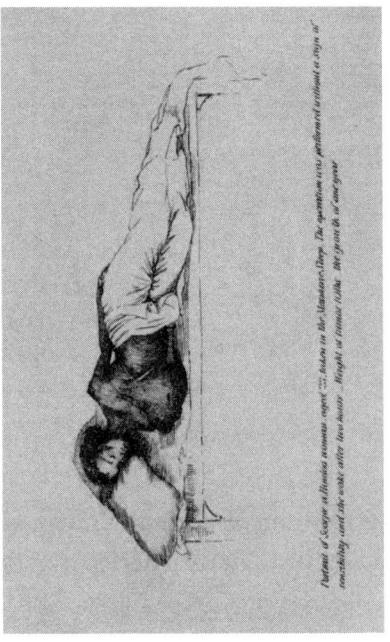

Source: *The Introduction of Mesmerism (with the Sanction of the Government) Into the Public Hospitals of India* by James Esdaile, M.D. Second Edition. W. Kent & Co. London, 1856.

Appendix 8

Title page of the book that contained a collection of letters relating to the work and progress of the Hooghly Imambarah (1815-1910). Published by Bengal Secretariat Book Depot, Calcutta in 1914.

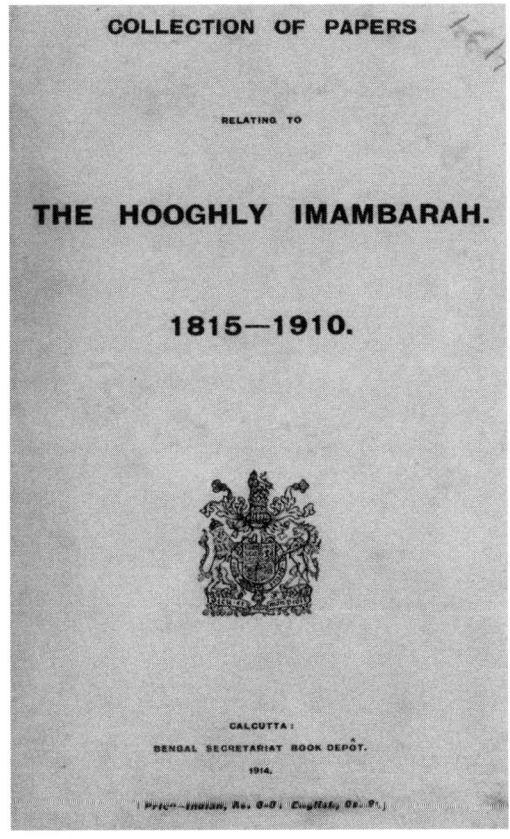

Appendix 9

Front page of the popular journal on mesmerism, *The Zoist: A Journal Of Cerebral Physiology & Mesmerism And Their Applications To Human Welfare*, edited by John Elliotson, published by Hippolyte Bailliere, London.

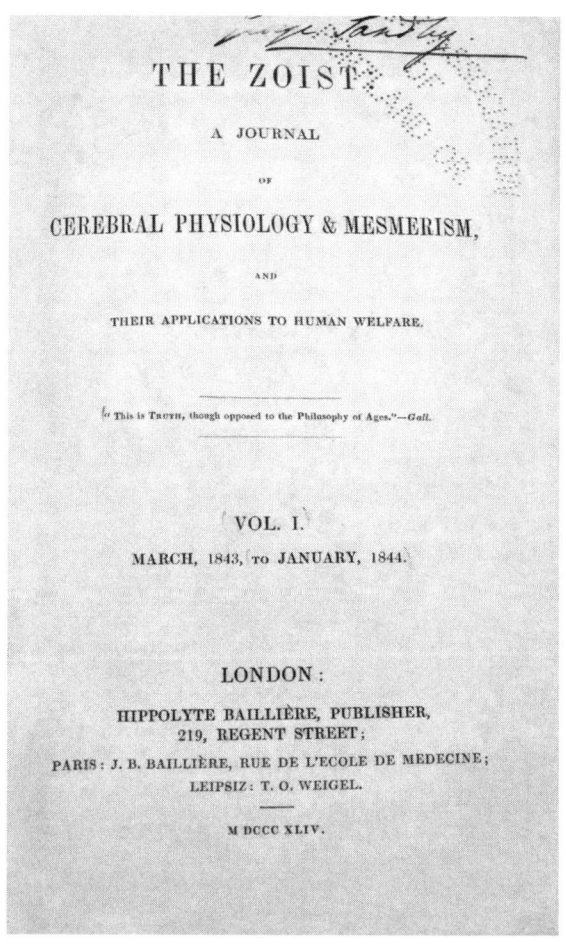

Appendix 10

Front page of James Esdaile's memoir, published from London in 1846.

MESMERISM IN INDIA,

AND ITS

PRACTICAL APPLICATION IN SURGERY AND MEDICINE.

BY

JAMES ESDAILE, M.D.

CIVIL ASSISTANT SURGEON, H.C.S. BENGAL.

"I rather choose to endure the wounds of those darts which envy casteth at novelty, than to go on safely and sleepily in the easy ways of ancient mistakings." — RALEIGH.

LONDON:
PRINTED FOR
LONGMAN, BROWN, GREEN, AND LONGMANS,
PATERNOSTER-ROW.
1846.

Appendix 11

Front page of the original report of Record of Cases Treated in the Mesmeric Hospital; From June To December 1847, Printed by Order of Government, Published from Military Orphan Press, Calcutta, 1848.

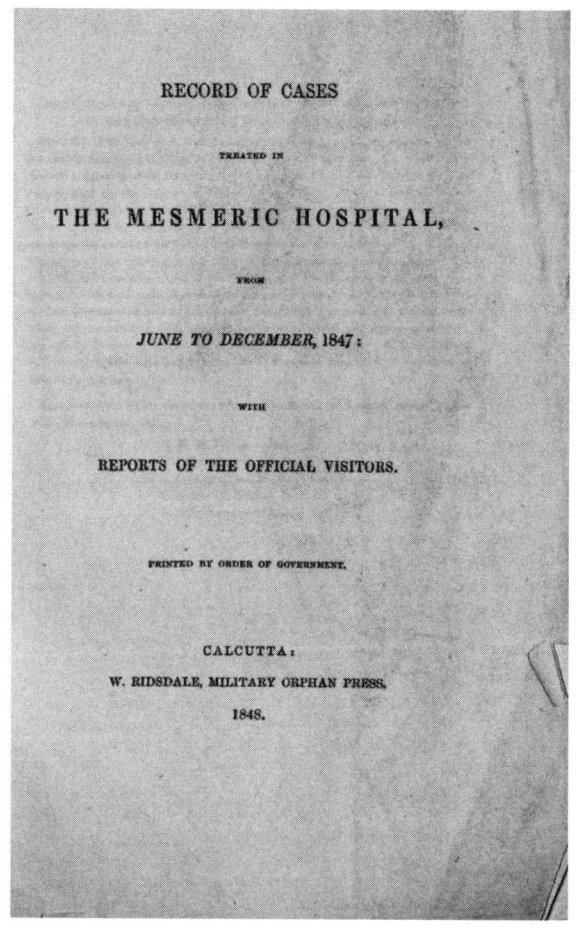

Appendix 12

Letters from Calcutta Mesmeric Hospital Visitors:

1. F.J. Mouat to W.M. Grey an officer undersecretary, Government of Bengal
2. From Medical Board Members including F. Hough, G. Lamb. To Honorable Sir T.H. Maddock, Deputy Governor of Bengal. 1847.

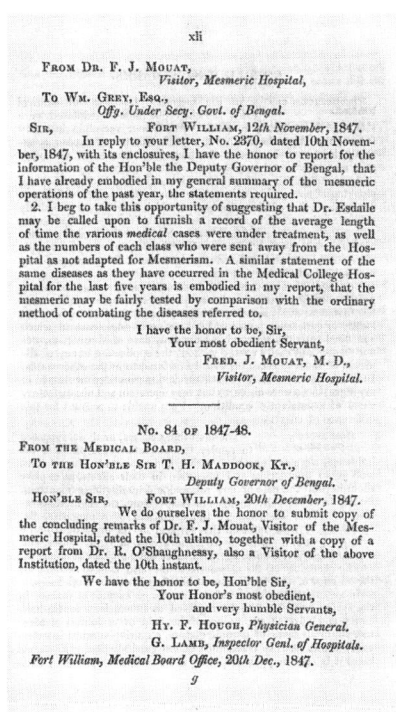

Source: *Record of Cases Treated in the Mesmeric Hospital; From June To December 1847,* Printed by Order of Government, Military Orphan Press, Calcutta, 1848, p. xli.

Appendix 13 A

Report of the Committee Appointed to Observe and Report on Dr. James Esdaile's Mesmeric Experiment – Submitted by Fred. Jas. Halliday, Secretary to the Government of Bengal, to J. Atkinson, Esq., Chairman, and W.B. O'Shaughnessy, Esq., Secretary of the Committee.

No. 2045.

TO J. ATKINSON, Esq., Chairman,
and
W. B. O'SHAUGHNESSY, Esq., Secretary of the Committee appointed to observe and report on Dr. Esdaile's Mesmeric Experiments.

GENTLEMEN,

Government of Bengal, Judicial—the 4th November 1846. I am directed to acknowledge the receipt of your letter dated the 9th ultimo, forwarding the Committee's Report, with Minutes of their proceedings and various documents referred to, the whole of which have been perused by the Hon'ble the Deputy Governor of Bengal with much interest and attention.

2. It appears from this Report that ten persons requiring Surgical treatment were subjected to the supposed mesmeric process; that of these, three were dismissed without effect, and the other seven patients, after various intervals, were thrown into a deep sleep, which however, according to the Committee, differed from natural sleep in as much as "the individual could not be aroused by loud noises; the pupils of the eyes were insensible to light; and great, and in some cases apparently perfect insensibility to pain was witnessed on burning, pinching and cutting the skin and other sensitive organs." On the other hand this sleep differed from that produced by narcotic drugs "in the quickness with which in eight cases out of ten the patient was awoke, after certain transverse passes, and fanning by the Mesmerizer, and blowing upon the face and eyes; in the natural condition of the pupils of the eyes and the conjunctiva in all the cases after awaking; in the absence of stertorous breathing, and of subsequent delirium, or hallucination, and of many other symptoms familiar to medical observers, and which are produced by Alcoholic liquors, Opium, Hemp, and other Narcotic drugs."

In the seven cases in which deep sleep was produced, operations were performed during this sleep; and the result is stated to be that three operations and one dressing were, to all appearance, perfectly painless; and in the other three there were "all the signs of intense pain which a dumb person might be expected to exhibit, except resistance to the Operator." "But," the Committee add, "in all these cases, without exception, after the operation was completed, the patients expressed no knowledge or recollection of what had occurred, denied having dreamed, and complained of no pain, till their attention was directed to the place where the operation had been performed." It appears from a table given by the Committee, and copied in the mar-

STATE OF PULSE.

Patient.	Disease.	Before.	During.	Imdly. after.	Operation.
Nilmoney, ..	Tumor, ...	84 ...	124	Natural,	Apparently painless.
Ditto, ...	Dressings changed on 12th September, ...	80 ...	108	Nat.,...	Apparently painless.
Domun, ...	Tumor, ...	72 ...	72	Nat.,...	Doubtful.
Jahirudin, ...	Excision of thickened prepuce ...	60 ...	60	Nat.,...	Doubtful.
Ramchund,..	Tumor, ...	68 ...	68	Nat.,...	Doubtful.
Hyder Khan,	Amputation of thigh, ...	108 ...	112	100	Apparently painless.
Murali Doss,	Tumor, ...	68 ...	108	72	Apparently painless.

gin, that the state of the pulse in these cases was not what might have been expected; being raised greatly in the apparently painless operations, and remaining unaffected in these which were accompanied by symptoms of pain.

"The general result arrived at, then," say the Committee, "on the question of pain during the Mesmeric Surgical Operations we witnessed, amounts to this, that in three cases there is no proof whatever that any pain was suffered, and that in three other cases the manifestations of pain during the operation are opposed by the positive statement of the patient that no pain was experienced."

Appendix 13 B

The Committee conclude their report by adverting to the necessity for an extensive, as well as accurate observation of the phenomena attending mesmeric agency, of the existence of which they seem to entertain little doubt. They attribute great merit to Dr. Esdaile for the "zeal, ability, and boldness with which he has taken up, and pursued this enquiry"; but they remark that his sphere has hitherto been limited, and they "hope that his further investigations may be extended to Medical, as well as Surgical, to European, as well as Native patients; and to the elucidation of the several questions which have been adverted to in the course of this Report."

3. The Deputy Governor concurs entirely with the Committee in thinking that though the investigations upon which their Report is founded have been upon a scale too confined to warrant any definite conclusion as to the existence and applicability of mesmeric agency to Surgical cases, yet the results hitherto observed are of sufficient importance to warrant a further prosecution of the enquiry. At the same time, His Honor is fully aware of the value of the time of the Members of the Committee, and that, as they have themselves observed, the responsible public duties on which most of the Members are employed, must suffer serious interruption, were the enquiry to be followed up under their observation, and *with equal strictness*, and to the requisite extent for the decision of the doubtful points they have indicated.

4. Under these circumstances, the Deputy Governor is unwilling to tax unnecessarily the time and convenience of the gentlemen forming the Committee; and in releasing them from the necessity of further attendance, I am instructed to convey the acknowledgments of the Government, and to express the satisfaction of the Hon'ble the President in Council as well as of the Deputy Governor of Bengal with the manner in which the Committee have performed their part in these important proceedings.

5. The Committee's Report has been ordered to be published, and the Deputy Governor entirely concurs with the remark of the President in Council, that it is sufficient for the present that it should be allowed to work its own way towards producing conviction among the profession and the public; and that, at this stage, any more direct encouragement on the part of Government to the general introduction of the mesmeric practice would be premature. But so far has the possibility of rendering the most serious surgical operations painless to the subject of them, been, in His Honor's opinion, established by the late experiments performed under the eye of a Committee appointed for the purpose, as to render it incumbent on the Government to afford to the meritorious and zealous officer by whom the subject was first brought to its notice such assistance as may facilitate his investigations, and enable him to prosecute his interesting experiments under the most favorable and promising circumstances.

6. With this view His Honor has determined, with the sanction of the Supreme Government, to place Dr. Esdaile for one year in charge of a small experimental hospital in some favorable situation in Calcutta, in order that he may, as recommended by the Committee, extend his investigations to the applicability of this alleged agency to all descriptions of cases, Medical as well as Surgical, and all classes of patients, European as well as Native. Dr. Esdaile will be directed to encourage the resort to his hospital of all respectable persons desirous of satisfying themselves of the nature and the effect of his experiments, especially Medical and Scientific individuals in or out of the Service; and His Honor will nominate from among the Medical Officers of the Presidency, "Visitors", whose duty it will be to visit the hospital from time to time, inspect Dr. Esdaile's proceedings, without exercising any interference, and occasionally, or when called on, report upon them, through the Medical Board, for the information of Government. On these Reports will mainly depend what further steps the Government may deem it expedient to take in the matter.

I have the honor to be,
Gentlemen,
Your most obedient Servant,
(Signed) FRED. JAS. HALLIDAY,
Secretary to the Govt. of Bengal.

W. RIDSDALE, BENGAL MILITARY ORPHAN PRESS.

Source: *The Original Report of The Committee Appointed by Government to Observe and Report upon Surgical Operation by Dr. J. Esdaile, Upon Patients Under The Influence of Alleged Mesmeric Agency,* Military Orphan Press, Calcutta, 1846. Collected from Wood Library Museum of Anesthesiology.

Appendix 14

A letter from James Esdaile to his father, 1st February 1846, Hooghly.

> TO THE
> ### REV. JAMES ESDAILE, D. D.
>
> My dear Father,
>
> However new and strange the subject of this work may be to you, I am sure that it will afford you pleasure to know that I have introduced, and I hope I may say established, a new and powerful means of alleviating human suffering among the natives of Bengal.
>
> I shall soon ascertain to what extent other varieties of mankind are capable of benefitting by this natural curative power, as I am ordered to join the army in the field, and depart to-morrow, by dâk, a journey of eleven hundred miles!
>
> I am
> Your affectionate Son,
> JAMES ESDAILE.
>
> HOOGHLY, Feb. 1st, 1846.

Source: *Mesmerism in India and Its Practical Application in Surgery and Medicine,* by James Esdaile (Silas Andrus and Son, New York, 1851).

Appendix 15

Franz Anton Mesmer, the Father of Mesmerism

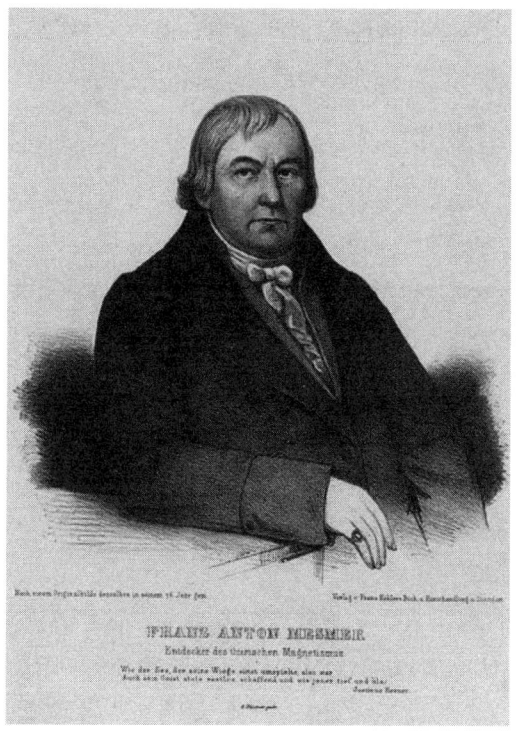

Source: *Mesmerism and the End of the Enlightenment in France* by Robert Darton (Cambridge: Harvard University Press, 1968).

Glossary

Company: East India Company

Hakeems: Practitioners of Unani medicine

Indigenous practitioners: Medicinal Practitioners of Ayurvedic and/or Unani medicine

State: The ruling government, the administrators

Vaids: Practitioners of Ayurvedic medicine

Western medicine: Medicine of the West (particularly of Britain). Or occidental medicine

Western practitioners: Practitioners of Western medical science

Babus or Bhadralok: Bengali elite to define for themselves a social class that would delineate their nobility

Ruqyah: It refers to the healing method based on the Quran and Hadith

Prophetic medicine: A genre of medical writing intended as an alternative to the exclusively Greek-based kind

Selected Bibliography

PRIMARY SOURCES

Gazetteers & Government Reports & Other Archival Documents

Archive, Index 133, Judicial Section, 138, 7th to 28th July, Proceeding 1847, 28/126, No 32, 7th July, BD/10, July/47, n 100, West Bengal State Archive.

Bengal and Agra (Miscellaneous). The Indian News, The Indian News and Chronicle of Eastern Affairs, London, 5th January 1849.

Bengal Past and Present, Journal of the Calcutta Historical Society, Volume 5, Part 1.

Collection Of Papers Relating To The Hooghly Imambarah 1815—1910, Calcutta, Bengal Secretariat Book Depot, 1914.

Collector of Customs, Financial Dept. Separate Revenue Branch, Gov. of Bengal.

Department of Revenue, Medical Branch, Gov. of Bengal.

Delhi Gazetteer, 24th December, 1846.

Deaths, The Asiatic Journal and Monthly Register for British and Foreign India, China, and Australasia, Volume 28, No. 110, February 1839.

Government Notifications: Civil and Ecclesiastical Appointments – Permanent, on 31 July 1849, *The Indian News and Chronicle of Eastern Affairs*, London, 5th January, 1849, p. 226.

GOI Medical, "GMC: A Report from the Pharmaceutical Committee on the Proposed Indian and Colonial Addendum to the BP of 1898" (March 1899), Asia, Pacific and Africa Collections, British Library (henceforth APAC), IOR/P/5645, pp. 373–97.

GOI Medical, "GMC: A Report from the Pharmaceutical Committee on the Proposed Indian and Colonial Addendum to the BP of 1898" (March 1899), Asia, Pacific and Africa Collections, British Welcome Library.

Gumming J. G. *Review of the Industrial Position and Prospects in Bengal in 1908*. Calcutta: 1908.

India Office. "Report of the Committee on the Supply of Drugs for India." 1875.

India Office. "Report of the Committee on the Supply of Drugs for India" (1875), APAC, IOR/L/MIL/7/15141.

Khambata, R.B. *Bengal Public Health Report of 1931*. Government of Bengal, Public Health Department, Bengal Secretariat Book Depot, 1933.

Medical Reporter: A Record of Medicine, Surgery, Public Health, and of General Medical Intelligence. Edited by Lawrence Frendandez, vol. II. Calcutta: The Medical Publishing Press, 1893.

Record of Cases Treated in The Mesmeric Hospital; From June to December, 1847, With Reports of Official Visitors, Printed by Order of Government. Calcutta: Military Orphan Press, 1848.

Record of Cases Treated in the Mesmeric Hospital; From June To December 1847, Printed by Order of Government. Calcutta: Military Orphan Press, 1848.

The Calcutta Journal of Medicine: A Monthly Record of The Medical and Auxiliary Science. Edited by Mahendralal Sircar, vol. XXIV. Calcutta: Anglo-Sanskrit Press, 1905.

The Calcutta Review, vol. XCVI, January 1893, Calcutta.

The London Medical Gazette, vol. IX, 6th September, 1851.

The Original Report of The Committee Appointed by Government to Observe and Report upon Surgical Operation by Dr. J. Esdaile, Upon Patients Under The Influence of Alleged Mesmeric Agency. Calcutta: Military Orphan Press, 1846. Collected from Wood Library Museum of Anesthesiology.

The Principles and Practice of Medicine; Founded on the Most Extensive Experience in Public Hospitals and Private Practice; and Developed in a Course of Lectures. Delivered at University College, London, by Dr. John Elliotson. London: Joseph Butler Medical Bookseller and Publisher, 1839.

The Reports of The Royal Commission of 1784 on Mesmer's System of Animal Magnetism and Other Contemporary Documents. English Translation by IML Donaldson (2014). Published for the James Lind Library and Royal College of Physicians of Edinburgh.

The Zoist: A Journal of Cerebral Physiology and Mesmerism and Their Application to Human Welfare. This journal appeared quarterly from April 1843 to December 1855. Total 13 volumes had been published.

West Bengal District Gazetteers, Hooghly. By Amya Kumar Benarji. Sree Saraswati Press, Calcutta. October 1972.

Crawford, Lt.-Colonel D. G. *A History of The Indian Medical Service 1600—1913*, Vol. Ii. London: W. Thacker & Co., 1914.

Memoirs, Autobiographies & Novels in English

Esdaile, James. *Mesmerism in India and Its Practical Application in Surgery and Medicine*. New York: Silas Andrus and Son, 1851.

———. "Mesmerism in The East." In *The Zoist* edited by John Elliotson, Vol. VII, March 1849 – January 1850. London: Hippolyte Bailliere.

Clarke, J.F. *Autobiographical Recollection of Medical Profession*. London: J & A Churchill, 1874.

Besant, Annie. *The Ancient Wisdom: An Outline of Theosophical Teachings*. London: [s.n.], 1890.

———. *Communication Between Different Worlds*. Adyar: [s.n.], 1913.

———. *Hypnotism and Mesmerism*. Adyar: Theosophical Publishing House, 1948.

Memoirs, Autobiographies & Novels in Bengali

Devi, Swarnakumari. "*Mesmerism ba Shaktichalana*." In *Bharati* (*Magh* 1292 Bengali Year or Jan.-Feb. 1886 CE).

———. "*Mesmerism ba Shaktichalana*." In *Bharati* (*Chaitra* 1292 Bengali Year or March-April 1886 CE).

———. "*Indriyer Sahajya Bina Moner Kotha Jana*." In *Bharati* (*Poush* 1291 Bengali Year or Dec. 1884 -Jan. 1885 CE).

Bandyopadhyay, Brojendranath. "*Jantob Chumbak-Shakti*." In *Bharati* edited by Swarnakumari Devi (*Magh* 1300 Bengali Year or Jan.-Feb. 1894 CE).

Bhattacharyya, Krishnakamal. "*Animal Magnetism ba Jantob Chumbak-Shakti*." In *Bharati* edited by Swarnakumari Devi (*Shraban* 1298 Bengali Year or July-August 1892 CE).

Chattopadhyay, Bankim Chandra. *Chandrashekhar*. Calcutta: Hare Press, 1897.

———. *Rajani*, Second Edition Calcutta: Bangadarshan Press, 1920.

Dutta, Ramesh Chandra. *Madhavi Kankan*. Kolkata: Annapurna Press, 1960.

Guha, Manoranjan. *Asha-Pradip*. Barishal: Manomohan Chakraborty, 1889.

Mukhopadhyay, Damodar. *Damodar Granthabali*, vol. 4. Calcutta: Purnachandra Mukhopadhyay.

Mukhopadhyay, Prabhat Kumar. "*Jogobal na Psychic Force.*" In *Prabhat Kumar Mukhopadhyayer Golpo Samagra*, vol. 4. Calcutta.

Shoka Vijaya. Calcutta: R.K. Mitter and Co., 1881.

Choudhurani, Saraladevi. *Jibaner Jharapata*. Sahitya Sangsad, 1879.

Newspapers & Magazines

Bengal Hurkaru, 1846, December.

Calcutta Morning Chronicle, 1851, December.

Ceylon Observer, 1846, November.

Ceylon Observer, 19 November, 1846.

"Painless Operations," *The Sydney Morning Herald*, Tuesday, 7 March 1848.

Pantha, Dwitiya Khanda, Nabya Parjya, Baishakh 1328, *Pratham Sangkhya*.

Sahitya Parishad Patrika, Poush – Magh 1295, Calcutta.

The Calcutta Star, 1846, November – December.

The Friend of India, 1846, November.

The Calcutta Star, 15 October 1846.

SECONDARY SOURCES

PhD Theses

Barik, Shaona. "Haunted by the Empire: Representations of the Occult and the Uncanny in Colonial Fiction about India, 1870-1940." Thesis submitted at Jadavpur University, Kolkata, 2018.

Basu, Anjali. "Bengal in the Reign of Aurangzib (1658-1707)." Thesis submitted at the University of London, School of Oriental and African Studies, London, 1965.

Basu, Ranu. "Urban Society in Bengal, 1850 – 1872, With Special Reference to Calcutta." Thesis submitted at School of Oriental Studies, University of London, 1974.

Basu, Mallika. "Science, Colonialism and Pharmaceutical Industries: Case Studies of Three Pharmaceutical Industries in Kolkata (1855-1947)." Thesis submitted at the Department of History, Vidyasagar University, 2013.

Basu, Shrimoye. "'Bazars' in the Changing Urban Space of Early Colonial Calcutta." Thesis submitted at the Department of History, University of Calcutta, 2015.

Chakravorty, Shreya. "Colonising the Body: Discourse of Mesmerism in Britain and Bengal, 1840-1900." Thesis submitted at Jadavpur University, Kolkata, 2018.

Chaudhuri, Shrimoy Roy. "Engrafting Modernity: Daktari in Nineteenth Century Bengal, c.-1830- c.1900." Thesis submitted at Syracuse University, December 2012.

Chakrabarti, Pratik. "Western Science and Modern India: Institutions, Individuals and Discourses." Thesis submitted at Jawaharlal Nehru University, New Delhi, 1999.

Mukharji, Projit Bihari. "Medicine and Modernity in Colonial Bengal: c. 1775 -1930." Thesis submitted at University of London, 2006.

Waltraud, R. M. Ernst. "Psychiatry and Colonialism: The Treatment of European Lunatics in British India, 1800-1858." Thesis submitted at The School of Oriental Studies, University of London, 1986.

Books in English

Arnold, David. *Colonising the Body: State Medicine and Epidemic Disease in Nineteenth Century India.* Delhi: Oxford University Press, 1993.

_____. *Western Medicine and Colonial India*, Vol-3. The New Cambridge History of India, Cambridge University Press, 2000.

_____, ed. *Warm Climates and Western Medicine, The Emergence of Tropical Medicine 1500-1900*, Clio Medica, The Wellcome Institute Series in the History of Medicine, Volume 35, Editions Rodopi, Brill, 1996.

_____, ed. *Imperial Medicine and Indigenous Societies.* Manchester: Manchester University Press, 1998.

Bala, Poonam. *Imperialism and Medicine in Bengal, A Socio historical Perspective.* New Delhi: Sage Publication, 1991.

Bandopadhyay, Arun, ed. *Science and Society in India, 1750-2000.* New Delhi: Manohar Publication, 2010.

Banerjee, Prajnananda. *Calcutta and Its Hinterland: A Study in Economic History of India, 1833-1900.* Calcutta: Progressive Publishers, 1975.

Bose, Pradip Kumar, ed. *Health and Society in Bengal: A Selection from Late 19th Century Bengal, A Periodical.* New Delhi: Sage Publication, 2006.

Caldwell, Charles. *Facts on Mesmerism and Thought on Its Causes and Uses.* Louisville, KY, 1842.

Chakrabarti, Pratik. *Western Science in Modern India, Metropolitan Method, Colonial Practice.* New Delhi: Permanent Black, 2004.

_____. *Medicine & Empire 1600 - 1960*. London: Palgrave Macmillan, 2014.

Chatterjee, Srilata. *Western Medicine and Colonial Society Hospital of Calcutta 1757-1860*. New Delhi: Primus Book, 2017.

Charles, Hall Radclyfe. *Mesmerism: its Rise, Progress, and Mysteries in all Ages and Countries: being a Critical Inquiry into its Assumed Merits and History of its Mock Marvels, Hallucinations, and Frauds*. New York: Burgess, Stringer and Co., 1845.

Crook, James R. *Hypnotism, How It is Done; It's Use and Dangers*. Boston: Arena Pub, 1894.

Das, Debanjani. *Houses of Madness Insanity and Asylums of Bengal in Nineteenth Century India*. New Delhi: Oxford University Press, 2015.

Elliotson, John. *Numerous Cases of Surgical Operation Without Pain In The Mesmeric State; With Remarks Upon The Opposition of Many Member of The Royal Medical And Chirurgical Society and Others to the Reception of The Inestimable Blessings of Mesmerism*. Philadelphia: Lea & Blanchard, 1843.

Esdaile, James. *Mesmerism in India and Its Practical Application in Surgery and Medicine*. New York: Hartford, Andrus and Son, 1851.

_____. *Natural and Mesmeric Clairvoyance with the Practical Application of Mesmerism in Surgery and Medicine*. London: H. Baillière, 1852.

_____. *The Introduction of Mesmerism, As an Anaesthetic and Curative Agent, into the Hospitals of India*. Perth: Printed for Dewar, 1852.

_____. *Hypnosis in Medicine and Surgery Creative Media Partners*. India: LLC, 1957.

Filenbrown, Thomas. *Hypnotism as Applied to Dentistry*. In *Dental Review*, Massachusetts, 1892.

Harrison, Mark. *Climates and Constitution; Health, Rave and British Imperialism in India 1600-1850*. New Delhi: 1999.

_____. *Public Health in British India, Anglo Indian Preventive Medicine, 1859-1914*. Cambridge: Cambridge University Press, 1994.

Kumar, Deepak. *Medicine and The Raj: British Medical Policy in India, 1835-1911*. New Delhi: Oxford University Press, 1998.

_____, ed. *Science and Empire Essays in Indian Context 1700-1947*. New Delhi: Anamika Prakashan, 1991.

_____*Unequal Contender, Unseen Ground Medical Encounter in British India 1820-1920 in Western Medicine as Contested Knowledge*. Edited by Biswamoy Pati and Mark Harrison. New Delhi: Orient Longman, 2001.

_____. *Disease & Medicine in India*. New Delhi: Tulika Books, 2012.

Mitter, Digammaber. *The Epidemic Fever in Bengal*. Calcutta: Hindon Patriot Press, 1876.

Mukharji, Projit Bihari. *Doctoring Traditions Ayurveda, Small Technologies and Braided Science*. Chicago: Chicago Press, 1916.

_____. *Nationalizing the Body: the Medical Market, Print and Daktari Medicine*. London: Anthem Press, 2009.

Pal, Dharma. *Indian Science and Technology in the Eighteenth Century; Some Contemporary European Accounts*. Academy of Gandhian Studies, India, 1983.

Rains, Geo. W. *Strange Forces In Nature and Their Relation To The Healing Art: An Introductory Lecture on the Course of 1874-75*. London: Jackson and Allis Street, 1874.

Raj, Kapil. *Colonial Encounters and The Forging of New Knowledge and National Identities, Great Britain and India, 1760-1850*. Oz iris, Vol. 15, 2000.

Roy, MacLeod, and Milton Lewis, ed. *Imperial Health in British India 1857-1900, in Disease, Medicine and Empire, Perspective on Western Medicine and The Experience of European Expansion*. London: Routledge, 2022.

Sandby, George, A. *Mesmerism And Its Opponents With A Narrative of Cases*. New York: Benjamin & Young, 1844.

Sen, Samita, and Anirban Das. "A History of The Calcutta Medical College and Hospital 1835-1936." In *Science and Modern India: An Institutional History, c.1784-1947, A Project of History of Science, Philosophy and Culture in Indian Civilization*, edited by Uma Dasgupta, Vol. XV, Part 4. Pearson India, 2010.

Townshend, Chauncey Hare. "Facts In Mesmerism With Reasons For A Dispassionate Inquiry Into It." New York: 1841.

Books in Bengali

Bagich, Ashok Kumar. *Chikitsa Swastha Yuge Yuge*. Calcutta: West Bengal State Book Board, 1984.

Chattopadhayaya, Biru. *Barania Biggyani Smarania Abiskar*. Barnali Prakakshani, 1982.

Dasgupta, Gyanendra. *Manashik Swastha*. Calcutta: Asiatic Book Agency, 1992.

Freud, Sigmund. *Swapna; Manaswikhan Bhumika*. Translated by A. Basu. Calcutta: 1997.

Gangopadhyaya, Dhirendranath. *Pabhlav Parichiti,* vol. 1-1957, vol. 2-1976. Calcutta: Mukherjee and Co.

Ghosh, Prabir. *Aloukik Noi Loukik*, vol. 2-1991. Calcutta: Dey's Publishing.

Rajendra, Rudra. *Sammohan Vidya*, Fourth Edition. Printed by Kalachand Basak, Narayan Machine Press, Calcutta, 1935. Digital Library of India, Item no, 2015.324521.

Paul, Arun Kumar. *Byatha Bedonar O Tar Upasham*. Calcutta: West Bengal State Book Board, 1986.

_____. *Anaesthesia*. Calcutta: West Bengal State Book Board, 1984.

Roy, Dilip Kumar. *Deshe Deshe Chali Ure*. Calcutta: Indian Associated Publishing Co. Ltd, 1954.

Sarkar, Sunil Kumar. *Freud*. Calcutta University, 1959.

Articles and Journals

Bhattacharya, Tinni Goswami. "Revisiting Health in Colonial Bengal: A Literary Overview (1880 –1930)." In *Journal of Social and Development Sciences*, Vol. 3, No. 11, Nov 2012.

Bhattacharya, Nandini. "Between the Bazar and the Bench: Making of the Drugs Trade in Colonial India, ca. 1900 – 1930." In *Bulletin of History of Medicine*, Vol. 90, No. 1, John Hopkins University Press, Spring 2016, pp. 61-91.

Chaudhuri, Runa Das. "Enchantingly Modern: Whispers of the Occult in Popular Psychic Healing Practices of Early 20th-century Bengal." In *The Oriental Anthropologist*, Vol. 21, No. 1, Sage Publication, 2021, pp. 86-103.

Crawford, D.G. *James Esdaile; Bengal Past and Present: Journal of the Calcutta Historical Society*, Volume 5, Issue 1, 1910.

Divekar, V.M., and L.D. Naik. "Evolution of Anaesthesia in India." In *Journal of Post Graduate Medicine*, Vol. 47, Issue 2, 2001, pp. 149-152.

Ernst, Waltraud. "Colonial Psychiatry, Magic and Religion. The Case of Mesmerism in British India." In *History of Psychiatry*, Vol. 15, Issue 1, 2004, pp. 57-71.

_____. "James Esdaile (1808–1859)." In *Oxford Dictionary of National Biography*, Oxford University Press, September, 2004.

_____. "'Under the Influence' in British India: James Esdaile's Mesmeric Hospital in Calcutta, and its Critics." In *Psychological Medicine*, Volume 5, Cambridge University Press, 1995, pp. 1113-1123.

———. "Beyond the East and West: From the History of Colonial Medicine to a Social History of Medicine in South Asia." In *Social History of Medicine*, Vol. 20, No. 3, 2007, pp. 505-524.

Gyan, Prakash. "Science 'Gone Native' in Colonial India." In *Representation*, No. 40, Special Issue, Seeing Science, University of California Press. Autumn 1992, pp. 153-178.

Kumar, Deepak. "Patterns of Colonial Science in India." *India Journal of History of Science*, Vol. 15, Issue 1, June 1980, pp. 105-13.

———. "The Culture of Science and Colonial Culture of India 1820-1920." *British Journal of History of Science*, Cambridge University Press, Vol. 29, Issue 2, June 1996, pp. 195-209.

Khandelwal, Sudhir. "Contributions of an Indian to the Science and Art of Hypnosis." In *Indian Journal of Psychiatry*, edited by Abbe Faria, Vol. 56, Issue 4, Oct.-Dec. 2014, p. 415.

Rajendran, Punnya. "Parrhesia and Clinical Practice: A Case Study of Dr. Esdaile's Mesmeric Hospital in Hooghly." In *Rupkatha Journal on Interdisciplinary Studies in Humanities*, Vol. 13, Issue 2, May 2021, pp. 1-13.

Raman, Ramya, and Anantanarayanan Raman. "Painless Surgery Joseph Johnstone Performed on a Mesmerized Patient in Madras in 1847." In *Indian Journal of History of Science*, Vol. 54, Issue 1, 2019, pp. 13-22.

Stephen, Leslie, ed. "James Esdaile." In *Dictionary of National Biography*, Vol. 18. Smith, Elder & Co., London: 1889.

Sharma, Vikash Kumar, Pranab Pandya, Gourab Gupta, Rakesh Kumar. "Evaluation of Hypnotherapy in Pain Management of Cancer Patients: A Clinical Trial from India." In *Indian Journal of Pain*, Vol. 31, Issue 2, 2017, pp. 100-106.

ACKNOWLEDGEMENTS

The inexorable pursuit of knowledge leads to the acquisition of rare and ancient records, preserved within the sanctums of the National Library in Calcutta and the West Bengal State Archive, where the eminent Bidisha Chakrabarty proves to be an invaluable guide. The unravelling of these hidden treasures enriches the tapestry of this study. I am also thankful to Dr Melissa Grafe, Head of the Medical Historical Library, Yale University, New Haven, United States, for providing me the last sixth month medical report of Mesmeric Surgery at the Calcutta Mesmeric Hospital. Without her contribution my project findings would be incomplete.

With profound gratitude, I extend my heartfelt appreciation to my esteemed supervisor Dr Arpita Sen whose unwavering support and guidance have been instrumental in bringing this book to fruition. To my father, Shankar Ghosal, and mother, Krishna Ghosal, I owe an immeasurable debt of gratitude for their belief in my potential and their constant encouragement. Furthermore, I express my deepest gratitude to my beloved wife Puja Chatterjee whose boundless love, illimitable and ceaseless encouragement have been a source of solace and motivation.

INDEX

A
Abdoolla, Sheik 128
Academy of Berlin, Germany 57
Academy of Sciences, Berlin 14
Ackley 17
Afzalganj Hospital, Hyderabad 135
Ali, Hakim 36
Ali, Muhammad 66
Allee, Syud Keramut 127
Altamish 35
American Society for Clinical Hypnosis 166
amputation 9, 52, 77, 89, 139
anaesthesia 10, 22, 56, 67, 120, 129, 137, 150, 170, 172, *see also* chloroform; ether gas
anaesthetic hypnosis: catalytic state or trance 53 (*see also* mesmeric trance); Hypnoidal 53; Lethargic State or Light Trance 53; Somnambulism 53, 67
anaesthetic surgery 21–22, 124, 152, 167, *see also* mesmeric surgery
Anderson, Captain 76
animal magnetism 10, 13–14, 16, 53–54, 56–57, 158, *see also* mesmerism
annals of surgical history 98
antecedent paroxysm 54
Asha Pradeep, Guha 162
Ashburner 124
asphyxia 138
Atkinson, J. 86–87, 90
Aurangzeb 29–30, 37
Australian Society for Clinical Hypnosis 166
Autobiographical Recollections of the Medical Profession, Clarke 21
Avicenna, Islamic physician 12
Ayurveda 29–38, 41–42, 44, 48, 154; in *Atre Samhita* or *Vela Samhita* 31; principles of 32; text translation into English 38; Trihumoral theory 179n23

B
babus 46–49, 122, *see also* class; elites
Bahadoor, Kalikishan, Rajah 126
Bahadur, Krishna, Raja 41
Bathgate and Co. 29
Battle of Plassey 39
bazaar medicines 141–42
Bengal Dispensatory and Pharmacopoeia O'Shaughnessy 124
Bengal Hurkaru 92, 122
Bengal Medical Service 39, 123–24
Bengal Pharmacopoeia, O'Shaughnessy 47
Bengalis 29, 144, 152, 159, 162, 170
Bentinck, William 42, 76, 138
Bernier, Francois 37
Besant, Annie 156, 158
bhadralok 122
Bhairon, Hakim 36
Bharati 158
Bhattacharya, Kunjabihari 165
Bhattacharya, Surendra Mohan 165
Bhowa, Mian 34
Bhuttacharge, Bonmallee (Banamali Bhattacharya) 97–98
Blavatsky, Helena Petrovna von Hahn 155–56
Blyth 127
Bodinier 17
Bose, Gopul Chunder 134
Bose, S.N. 165
Bostwick 17
Botanical Observations on Selected Indian Plants, Jones 40

Brahminism 33
Braid, James 15, 57, 157–58, 161
Bramley, M.J. 42, 44
The British Chemical Works 29
British Medical Association 136; Glasgow Committee 136
British Society of Clinical and Academic Hypnosis 166
Buddhism, Vinaya Pitaka 33
Butcher 127
Buttokrishno Paul and Co. 29

C
C. Ringer and Co. 29
Calcutta Medical and Physical Society 41
Calcutta Medical College (CMC) 38, 43–46, 119, 124, 141, 153, 163
Calcutta Medical Journal 19, 101
Calcutta Medical School 154
Calcutta Mesmeric Hospital 19–20, 23, 60–62, 64, 93, 95, 100, 103, 108–9, 119–21, 123, 145, 147, 152–53, 173; ambivalence in 121–23; birth of 90, 93; closure of 145
Campbell Medical School, Sealdah 46
carbonic acid gas 10
case reports 84, 101, 111–18
Chakrabarti, Pratik 25
Chakroborty, Kshitish Chandra 165
Chandrashekhar, Chattopadhyay 159–61
Charak Samhita 33
Charaka 31, 42
Chatterjee, T.H. 127
Chattopadhyay, Bankim Chandra 159, 161
Chenevix, Richard, Irish doctor 58
chloroform 9–10, 19–20, 52, 135–40, 145, 150–53, 167; adverse outcomes of 150; anaesthesia 134–37; Bennett on 138; death by 136, 138–39; first use of 134; phased out 136
'Chloroformed' 137
Choudhury, J. 165
Chowdhury, Subarna Roy 30
The Christian Advocate 121
Christie, R. 63
Clark, John 40
Clarke, J.F. 21

class 164; aristocratic 163; Bengali LMS 46; English-speaking 141, 154; middle 47–48, 125, 141, 143, 164; upper 143; wealthy 126
Clinical and Applied Hypnosis at Saybrook University in UK 166
clinical hypnosis 56
Clinical Illustrations of the More Important Diseases of Bengal, Twining 40
Cloquet, Jules 58
Colebrook, Major 131
Colonial Bengal 39, 45, 134, 151, 167; mesmerism in 10
colonialism 15–16, 48
consciousness 53, 72, 96–97, 102, 109
Copland 50
Cordon, Evelyn 127
Cornwallis, Lord 40
courses: Doctor of Medicine (MD) 46; M.A. Specialization in Parapsychology 166
Cowasji, Rustomjee 163
Currie, Sir F. 131

D
Dalhousie, Lord 19, 64, 119–22
Darush-Shifa 37
Date, Dr 137
Day, Rajani Kanta 45
De, Rajkrishna 45
De imperio solis ac lunae in corpora humana, et morbis inde oriundis, Mead 55
De Narcotics ('On Narcotics') 63
Deb, Promothonath (Promoth Nath Dev) 126
Delafield, Francis 17
Delson, M. 56
Dev, Radhakanta, Rajah 41, 125–26
Dhanvantari 31, 33, *see also* Ayurveda
disease: bladder rupture 69; blindness 13, 164; body trembled 131–32; broken right wrist 129–30; bursa enlargement 105–6; colis 129; dyspepsia 164; fever 27, 69, 78, 104, 150; headaches 12, 132; heart problems 164; hernia 68; hypertrophied scrotum 106; hysteria

13, 143, 164; malaria 164; menstrual irregularities 164; mental illnesses 164; mute 130; nervous and vascular systems 147; nervous headaches 71; paralysis 13, 100, 132, 164; rheumatism 86, 99–100, 102, 105, 109, 131, 164; scirrhous testes 9, 106; severe fever and nervous headaches 105; sleeplessness 164; stiff in left elbow 99; stiff in joints 131–32; swollen hands 132; toothaches 164
dispensaries 47, 154
Dissertatio Physico-Medica de Planetram in fluxu, Mesmer 54
drugs, imported 29, 47, *see also* medical market, Calcutta
Ducas 17
Dutt, Rameshchandra 159–60
Dutta, Chakrapani 31

E
Early Remedies 30–37
East India Company 17, 29–30, 41, 44, 46, 62–63, 128, 145, 152
Eckford, Brigadier 131
economic crisis 133
Eden Hospital, Calcutta 47
Edlin 127
Edward, Ives 26–27, 163
Eggerton 44
Electric Telegraphy 124
electric torpedo fish 12
Electroencephalograms (EEGs) 52
elites 122, 125–26, 133, 145, 153, 163, *see also* class
Elliot, H.M. 19, 126
Elliotson, John 15, 23, 57–60, 82, 84, 124, 127, 133–34, 161
Engledue 127
epilepsy 13, 106; cure 109
Ernst, Waltraud 23
Esdaile, James (Scottish Civil Surgeon) 17–20, 22–23, 51, 57–58, 60–61, 62–74, 76–9, 82–93, 95–96, 100–104, 108, 118–25, 127–34, 137, 139–40, 143–46, 152, 155, 161, 170, 173; articles by 23; as Calcutta Presidency Surgeon 119; death of 127; first painless surgical operation of 18; as 'Jadoowala' 22; report to *The Englishman* 82
ether gas 10, 19–21, 52, 124, 136–38, 146, 149–51
European Society of Hypnosis 166
Ezra Hospital, Calcutta 47

F
Facts in Mesmerism with Reasons for a Dispassionate Inquiry into It, Townshend 22
Fa-Hien 33
Ferdunji, Rupbai, first anaesthetist in India 136
Fisher, H., Rev 19, 70–72, 126
Fitzpatrick 127
Foissac, M. 14
Forbes, John 19
Fractured Foundations 133–34
Francis, John W. 17
Franklin, Benjamin 57

G
Gandhi, Mahatma 136–37
Ganges 27
Ghosain, Nufferloll 134
Ghosal, Janakinath 157
Ghosal, Sutt Churn, Rajah 19
Ghosal, Swarnakumari Devi 156–58
Ghose, Ramgopal 19, 126–27
Glover, Robert Mortimer 10
Goodeve 44
Gordon, Alice 156
Gordon, E.M. 87
Gosaul, Rajah Suttuchurn 126
Grant, A. 127
Grant, John 42
Great Revolt of 1857 46
Greek medical systems 32
Guha, Manoranjan 162
Guillotine 56–57
Gupta, Dwaraknath 45
Gupta, Madhusudan 41, 45

H
Haji Muhammad Mohsin 18
hakims 34, 37, 154

Halliday, F.J. 90
Hamilton, Alexander 39
Hasim, Mir Muhammad, Hakim 37
healing pattern, pre-colonial 30–37
healthcare 28, 33–34, 37, 166, 170–73; institutions 167; professionalization of 170, 172; professionals 164
Heatly 127
Hedges, William 29
Hehir, Patrick 135
Hell, Maximilian 13, 56
herbal remedies 170
Hooghly Charity and Jail Hospital 84
Hooghly Imambarah Hospital: or Hazi Muhammad Mohsin Hospital 18, 51, 62–63, 65, 76, 79, 157; first painless surgical operation 18; mesmeric surgery at 19; Mohsin Fund of 18
Hooghly Jail Hospital 19, 62–65, 71, 84
Hooghly Native Hospital 87
Hooghlyr Imambari, Swarnakumari Devi Ghosal 157
hospital medicine 155
Hough, Major 127
Hume, James 19, 92, 125–27
Hume, J.A.S. 87
Hyderabad Chloroform Commissions (First and Second) 135–36
hypnoidal 53
hypnosis/hypnotism 23, 17, 51–52, 57, 70, 155–58, 160–61, 165, 167; in modern medical science 58; Mukhopadhyay on 160
hypnotherapy 51

I
illnesses 28, 52, 93, 165; equipments for 165
imperialism 48, 167
Indian medical system 38, 41, 43, 154
indigenous medical system 38, 47, *see also* ayurveda; herbal remedies; Unani medicine
'*Indriyer Sahajya Bina Moner Kotha Jana*' (Mind-Reading Without Sensory Assistance), Swarnakumari Devi 157

J
Jackson, J. 87
Jackson, J.J. 87
Jainism 33
Jibaner Jharapata, Chaudhurani 162
Jivaka of Magadha 31, 33
Jogobal na Psychic Force? 160
Johnson, Joseph 18
Jones, William 40

K
kabirajs/Kavirajas 34, 48 39
Kashyap Samhita, Jivaka 31
Kemp, A. 127
Keora, Madhav (Madhab Keora) 65–67
Khalji, Mahmud 35
Khan, Ajmal, Hakim 154
Khan, Ibrahim 30
Khan, Salahuddin Muhammad, founder of Hooghly Imambarah 18
Khan, Shaista 29
Khanum, Zainab 17
Koochill, Shaik 96–98
Krishna, Rajah Kali 19

L
La Croix, Rev. 19, 126, 140
The Lancet 27, 60
Largus, Scribonius 12
Lawrie, Edward 135–36
Levsier 57
'Licentiates in Medical and Surgery' (LMS) 46
Liston, Robert 60
Littler, John, Sir 19, 131
Louis XVI 12, 56

M
Macaulay Minutes 43
Madame 58
Maddock, Herbert, Sir 19, 137
Maden-Ush-Shifa Tibbe Sikender Shahi, Bhowa 34
Madhavi Kankan, Dutt 159
Magnes 11
Magnesia 11

Index

magnetic: stones 11; therapy 11–12; treatments 12
magnetism 11–13, 54–57
Mahetie, Sonatun 96, 98
Majmua-i-Ziae 36
Marcel, French physician 12
Martin 19, 126–28, 140
Maxwell, William 11
Mayow, Captain 131
Mead, Richard 54–55
Medical Act 46
medical care 10, 35; palliative or 10
medical college 42–43, 45–47, 65, 119, 149
Medical College Hospital, Calcutta 43, 135
medical market, Calcutta 163
Medical Registration Acts 164
medical science 9, 30, 32, 36, 40–41, 46, 48, 50–51, 101, 119, 169
medicinal plants 28, 142, *see also* herbal remedies
Menace, Niocolao 37
Mesmer, Franz Anton, or Frederick Anthony Mesmer 11–13, 16, 51, 58, 170, 205; on anaesthetize 56; animal magnetism 57, 157; death of 57; energy and magnet 55
mesmeric anaesthesia 18–24, 59–60, 62, 65, 67–68, 79, 82, 87, 124, 127, 144, 146, 153, 172–73 (*see also* mesmeric trance; mesmerism); first applied 58; healing or treatment 99, 102, 109; intervention 101–3; institutionalization of 170–71; resurgence of 163–67; visitors' chronicles 123–24
Mesmeric Hospital, Calcutta 11, 23–24, 92, 98, 106, 121–23, 125–27, 130, 133, 138, 144–45; as 'Jadoo Hospital' 21–22
mesmeric surgery 57–62, 59, 90, 93–110, 119, 127, 140, 142; as painless 18, 20, 24, 48, 51, 60, 62–63, 64–65, 86, 90, 120, 124, 136
mesmeric trance 62, 64, 69, 71, 84, 86, 97, 99–100, 102–3, 106, 119, 122, 140, 143, 146; Chattopadhyay on 159
mesmerism 10, 19, 22–23, 61, 83, 139, 157 (*see also* mesmeric anaesthesia); in Bengali Literature 158–62; Birth of 11–21; cessation of 137, 145, 174; Dutt on 159; factors against 153–54; and hypnotic application 164; integrating in surgery 15, 48, 149; and medical ethics 148; Mukhopadhyay on 160, 160–61; sanctity of 144–51; and Science 51–57; treatment without surgery 132
Mesmerism in Colonial India, Esdaile 9
Mesmerism in India, Elliotson ed. 23
Mesmerism in India and its Practical Application in Surgery and Medicine, Esdaile 22
mesmerism movement 14–21, 61
Messrs. H.M. Elliott 127
Mitra, Nabin Chandra 45
Mitter, Ramchunder 127
modern hypnotism 53
modernity 44, 142, 144, 153, 172; mystique and 144–51
Mohsin, Muhammad 17
mortality rates 27–28
Motahar, Agha Muhammad 17
Mott, Valentine 17
Mouat, J.F. 94, 108, 123, 125, 147
bin Muhammad, Yusuf, Hakim 36
Mukherjee, Sujata 38
Mukhopadhyay, Damodara 162
Mukhopadhyay, Prabhat Kumar 160–61

N

National College of Hypnosis and Psychotherapy, UK 166
nationalist movement (swadeshi) 141, 154, 157, 163–64
Nationalist Surge 155
Native Medical Institutions (NMI) 41–43
naval medical care 26
Neuralgia 132
neuro-hypnotism ('sleep of the nerves') *see* hypnotism/hypnosis
nitric acid 52
nitrous oxide or laughing gas 10
non-cooperation movement 163
Numerous Cases of Surgical Operation Without Pain in The Mesmeric State, Elliotson 22, 59

O

observational medicine 155–58, 163
Observations on the Diseases which prevail in the Long Voyages to Hot Countries, Clark 40
occultism 143, 147
Olcott, Henry Steel, Col. 155–56, 158
'On Death from Chloroform,' Sibson on 138
opium dependence 129
O'Shaughnessy, R. 44, 94, 149–50
O'Shaughnessy, W.B. 44, 47, 87, 90, 123
Ovingto, Johan 38

P

pantomime 130
Paracelsus 12
Paré, Ambroise 10
Paris Medical Society 10
Patronage of Mesmeric Healing by elites of Calcutta 125–33
Pavlov, Ivan Petrovich 52
Pharmacopoeia of India 46
Physick, Philip Syng 10
Poyen, Charles 16
A Practical Account of the Epidemic Cholera, Twining 40
Praksha, Bhaba 42
Prasad, Jyoti 137
The Principles and Practice of Medicine, Elliotson 59
pseudoscience 162, 165
psychic: healers 162, 164–65; healing 164, 166
psychotherapy 160
Puysegur at Busancy 53

Q

quack doctors 48

R

Rajani, Chattopadhyay 159, 161
Rajendran, Punnya 23
Al-Razi 32
Regulating Act of 1773 30
Riddell, Major 76
Rogers, A. 87
Rosen, George 24

Ross, James Clark 79
Roy, Nundkishore (Nanda Kishore Roy) 93–95, 127
Roy, Rama Persaud 19, 126
Roy, Buddhinath, Raja 163
Roy, Kumar Kalikrishna 127
Roy, Madan Mohan 73, 127
Roy, Modoosooden 127
Roy, Nursing Chunder, Rajah 126, 163, 165
Roy, Rammohun 134
Roy, Ramprashad 127
Royal Commission, France 12, 56
Royal Medical and Chirurgical Society, London 50, 57, 59
Rudra, Rajendranath 165
Rustamji 135

S

Salahuddin, Mannoojan Khanum 18
Saleh, Muhammad, as Salah Uddin Muhammad Khan 17
Sanjak, Hakim 37
Sannud, Abdool 127
Sanskrit College, hospital for Western medicine with 42–43
Saraladevi Chaudhurani 162
Sarkar, Jadunath 29
Sayers, Captain 131
Seal, Motilall (Motilal Shill) 126
Seebchunder, Raja 163
Sein, Hurrymohun (Hiraanmoy Sen) 127
Sen, Ram Comul 41–42, 163
Set, Purmanund 134
Set, Umacharan 45
Shakha Vijay, Mukhopadhyay 161
Shambhunath Pandit Hospital in Bhabanipur 47
Shifa-khana 35
Shukalbasona Sundari, Mukhopadhyay 162
Shyama Charan Laha Eye Hospital, Calcutta 47
Sibson 138, 150
Sidney, A. 17
Simpson, James Y. 10, 134
Sing, Pertub Chunder, Rajah 19, 126
Sircar, Isser Chunder 134
Sissmore, Charles T. 79

Index

Society for Psychical Research 158
Spens, Thomas 42
spiritualism 155, 158
St. Thomas Hospital 60
stethoscope, discovery of 57, 59
Stewart, D. 87, 90, 138
Strong's insane asylum 132
Suja, Shah 29
Sukeahs Lane Hospital & Dispensary 19–20, 127, 133–34
sulphuric ether gas. *See* ether gas
superstition 143, 145, 147, 153
surgical: interventions 74, 77, 79, 104, 106, 128, 149, 151; operations 10, 23, 63, 67, 9, 82, 87, 89, 124
Sushruta, physician 9, 31–32, 42
Sushruta Samhita 31
Sutherland, J.C.C. 79

T

Tagore, Debendernauth (Debendranath Tagore) 126–27
Tagore, Ramanoth 126–27, 156
Tagore, Devendranath 156
Tagore, Dwarakanath 163
Tahir, Shaikh Muhammad 36
Theosophical Society 152, 157; in Calcutta 156; and mesmerism 155–58; in New York 155
Thompson 93
Thomson 146
Thomson, James 131
Thomson, Scott 127
Trevelyan, C.E. 42
Tubbs, W.J. 21
Tughlaq, Firuz Shah 35
tumour 9, 85, 89, 94–95, 103–4, 106–7, 110, 131 (*see also* diseases); of 103 lbs 90; breast 58, 130; cartilaginous 95; cranium 93; in eye 128; in groin 78; hypertrophic scrotal 98; maxillary antrum 74; over cheek-bone 75; of right mamma 70; scrotal 84, 86, 90, 96–98, 101–2, 104, 106–10, 129; of seventy pounds 130; testicular 128
Twining, William 40

U

Uah, Hajee Faizu 17; marrying, Zainab Khanum 17–18
Unani medicine 29, 31, 37, 44, 46, 48
Unani Tibb 37

V

vaidyas 34–35, 37, 154, *see also* kabirajs
Van Helmont 11
Vernacular Licentiate in Medical Service (VLMS) 154

W

W. Markillical and Co. 29
Wagentreiber 127
Wakley, Thomas 19
Waldie, David 135
Wallich 44
Wars, 26; First World 164
Watson, Admiral 28
Webb, Alan 127, 131–32, 134
Western: ascendancy 141–43; capitalism 145; civilising mission 142; drug market 141–42; imperialism 145, 153; medical disciplines 44; medical mastery 42–49; medical science 29, 49, 45, 51, 148, 167; trained doctors 148
Western medicines 28–29, 38–40, 43, 45, 47, 49, 67, 141–42, 154, 172–73; in Bengal 37–42; as 'Colonial Enclaves' 141; market 153; mesmerism and 167, 169; rise of 134–43
Western pharmaceutical industry 141–42, 153
Westernization 29, 48
Wheelock 17
Wilby 127
Wilkinsons 29
Wise, T.A. 18
witchcraft 147, *see also* superstition

Z

zamindars 37, 46
The Zoist 23, 58, 60, 84, 124; 'An Account of the Mesmeric Hospital in Bengal since Dr. Esdaile's Departure from India' in 134